W0234928

Ethics and the Good Doctor

Ethics and the Good Doctor brings together existing literature and an analysis of empirical research conducted by the Jubilee Centre for Character and Virtues to examine the ethical nature of medical practice and explore medicine as a virtuous profession.

The book is based on the idea that medical practice is an inherently moral profession, in which notions of trust, care and meaningful relationships form the foundations of being a good doctor. By taking into account the ethical dimensions of medical practice that have come under greater scrutiny and pressure over recent years, this book explores how personal and professional character is understood, enacted, and experienced by medical practitioners at various stages of their career.

Ethics and the Good Doctor situates and presents the empirical data in a way that is accessible to practicing doctors, medical students, and medical educators. Clear implications for policy, practice, and research are offered, ensuring this book will be of great interest to a range of stakeholders involved in medical practice, including those working in medical policy.

Sabena Jameel is a General Practitioner (family medicine) and is also Quality Lead and Medical Professionalism Lead for the University of Birmingham Medical School, UK.

Andrew Peterson is Professor of Character and Citizenship Education and Deputy Director of the Jubilee Centre for Character and Virtues at the University of Birmingham, UK.

James Arthur is Professor of Education and Civic Engagement and Director of the Jubilee Centre for Character and Virtues at the University of Birmingham, UK.

Character and Virtue Within the Professions
Series Editors
James Arthur, *Professor of Education and Civic Engagement and Director of the Jubilee Centre for Character and Virtues at the University of Birmingham, UK.*

Andrew Peterson, *Professor of Character and Citizenship Education and Deputy Director of the Jubilee Centre for Character and Virtues at the University of Birmingham, UK.*

The principal objective of the series is to highlight the interplay between practitioners' personal character and the ethical dimensions of their professional domain. Each book will explore the specific ethical dimensions of the given profession at hand, including the interplay between professionals' individual character virtues and their working environments. In a time when cultures of managerialism, auditing, performance metrics and commercial success are seemingly increasing, this series attempts to re-focus the professions towards the ethical and societal origins that each profession intends to serve. Underpinned by perspectives of philosophy, psychology and sociology, each book will offer practitioners fresh viewpoints about how their character and professional context can influence their professional practice.

Books in the series include:

Ethics and the Good Teacher
Character in the Professional Domain
Andrew Peterson with James Arthur

Ethics and the Good Doctor
Character in the Professional Domain
Sabena Jameel, Andrew Peterson and James Arthur

For more information about this series, please visit:
www.routledge.com/Character-and-Virtue-Within-the-Professions/
book-series/CVP

Ethics and the Good Doctor

Character in the
Professional Domain

**Sabena Jameel, Andrew Peterson
and James Arthur**

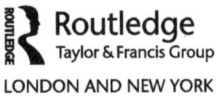

Routledge
Taylor & Francis Group

LONDON AND NEW YORK

First published 2022
by Routledge
2 Park Square, Milton Park, Abingdon, Oxon OX14 4RN

and by Routledge
605 Third Avenue, New York, NY 10158

Routledge is an imprint of the Taylor & Francis Group, an informa business

British Library Cataloguing-in-Publication Data
A catalogue record for this book is available from the British Library

Library of Congress Cataloging-in-Publication Data
A catalog record has been requested for this book

ISBN: 978-0-367-68511-9 (hbk)
ISBN: 978-0-367-68512-6 (pbk)
ISBN: 978-1-003-13788-7 (ebk)

DOI: 10.4324/9781003137887

Typeset in Times New Roman
by Newgen Publishing UK

Contents

Acknowledgements

This book is the second in a series of texts that examine *Character and Virtues in the Professions.* Each book in the series is dedicated to a specific profession and brings together reviews of existing literature and sources of empirical data – including data collected in various projects by the Jubilee Centre for Character and Virtues – to provide new insights for both pre- and in-service professionals, as well as acting as an educational resource to inform future professional decision-making and practice.

As we make clear from the outset, this book draws extensively on data and analysis from one of a number of research projects on virtues in the professions conducted and reported on by the Jubilee Centre that were all led by the Centre's Director, James Arthur. For this reason, we owe our sincere gratitude to those colleagues whose data collection, analysis, recommendations and overall insight on the project, including in the resulting report, has made this book possible. In particular, our thanks and acknowledgements go to Kristján Kristjánsson, Hywel Thomas, Ben Kotzee, Agnieszka Ignatowicz and Tian Qiu. We are also grateful to our colleagues at Routledge – in particular Anna Clarkson, Sarah Hyde and Will Bateman – for their interest and support in this series and book.

Sabena Jameel
Andrew Peterson
James Arthur

Introduction

Introduction

This book, and the main study from which the data contained within it is drawn, are premised on the idea that what constitutes a 'good' doctor necessarily involves more than technical skills and medical knowledge. While it would not make sense to conceive of a good doctor who does not possess the requisite medical knowledge and technical skills, what patients often desire from their doctors – and indeed what doctors often expect of themselves – is a professional who cares, who is compassionate, who empathises, and who they can trust to make an informed judgement. Professional qualities have long been at the heart of the medical profession, and are often framed in some way or other within key documents underpinning medical education. The General Medical Council's *Generic Professional Capabilities Framework* and *Outcomes for Graduates* documents, for example, structures the outcomes expected of medical school programmes around three categories – 'professional values and behaviours', 'professional skills', and 'professional knowledge' (GMC, 2017, 2018). Moreover, of all the professions within and without those specifically concerned with healthcare, it is the medical profession that we place the highest ethical expectations on (Paterson, 2013). Because of the intimate relationship between a doctor and their patients, trust is vital, particularly given that at key moments, lives, and indeed the quality of lives, are literally in the hands of doctors. It is perhaps for this reason that public shock and anger is so fervent and passionate when doctors transgress the trust invested in them.

Recognising that medical practice involves an ethical dimension and represents an essentially moral undertaking is one thing; explicating the precise nature of this ethical and moral dimension is another, and perhaps more difficult and contentious, matter. As we examine in later chapters, a large body of literature now exists that considers the moral

DOI: 10.4324/9781003137887-1

work of doctors, including how workplace environments and healthcare systems impact on such work. In this regard, the medical profession is not unique, with broadly comparable interest also evident in the moral dimensions of a number of professions. Yet, as is increasingly attested in the available literature and as is often featured across public media, over the last several decades the work of doctors has become more and more influenced by the pressures of market logic and, to some extent, regulatory accountability. To put it simply, doctors' work in environments in which meeting externally set targets, allocating limited resources, and increasing need for such resources, all place significant pressures on doctors' ability to enact their moral qualities. These pressures, in turn, contribute to pressures on retention, with a recent rapid review of the 'workforce crisis in medicine' identifying concerns around 'low morale', 'disconnect' between doctor and patient expectations, 'unmanageable change', and lack of personal and professional support' (Andah et al., 2021: 4–5; see also West and Coia, 2019).

The giving of serious attention to medical ethics curriculum in the UK can be traced to the Institute of Medical Ethics' (IME) *Pond Report on the Teaching of Medical Ethics* (Institute of Medical Ethics, 1987) and to the GMC's report *Tomorrow's Doctors: recommendations on undergraduate medical education* (1993) that contained much on education in ethics and professionalism. In 1998, the IME and GMC worked together to develop a model core curriculum for teaching medical ethics and legal issues to undergraduate medical students (Ashcroft et al., 1998). Notably, given our interest here in virtue-based approach to professional ethics, in the 2009 iteration of the core curriculum, the words 'character' and 'virtue' were not mentioned at all, but were alluded to in references to 'skills, attitudes and behaviours'. Following a review in 2017–2018, a further revised core curriculum was published in 2019 with the aim to 'equip students to identify ethical and legal issues in medical practice, have a critically reflective approach to those issues, and be able to give a reasoned justification of the actions they would take in line with the knowledge, attitudes and skills in the rest of this document' (IME, 2019: 2). Again, the terms 'character' and 'virtue' do not feature explicitly in the curriculum. Nor, for that matter, do the concepts of 'judgement' and 'wisdom'. Under the heading of 'professionalism', the curriculum advocates that students should be able to:

- Critically examine and apply General Medical Council guidance, principally relating to- the need to promote best practice and respect for patients, colleagues, and other healthcare professionals

- professional standards expected of students
- respecting the different beliefs of patients, students and other
- duty of candour
- maintaining professional boundaries with patients
- conscientious objection and its limits
- potential conflicts of interest use of social media
- Discuss the importance of trust, integrity, honesty and accountability in all professional relationships
- Recognise the limitations of their practical skills and knowledge, and to know how and where to seek appropriate sources of support [including when working abroad or in resource-poor environments]
- Identify and appropriately respond when there is cause for concern, when things could be improved, and when they go wrong
- Apply professional guidance across all clinical contexts, including while working abroad and in resource poor environments
- Consider the extent to which expected professional conduct extends into private life.

(IME, 2019: 7)

In somewhat of a contrast, the General Medical Council's *Generic Professional Capabilities Framework* emphasises a more developed and detailed conception of professional values and behaviours. While the terms 'character' and 'virtues' are not used explicitly (character and virtue do not necessarily align easily with educational frameworks that are easily mapped to codified competencies and assessment), under the domain of professional values and behaviours the following are expected:

- acting with honesty and integrity
- maintaining trust by showing respect, courtesy, honesty, compassion and empathy for others, including patients, carers, guardians and colleagues
- treating patients as individuals, respecting their dignity and ensuring patient confidentiality
- taking prompt action where there is an issue with the safety or quality of patient care, raising and escalating concerns where necessary
- demonstrating openness and honesty in their interactions with patients and employers – known as the professional duty of candour

- being accountable as an employee to their employer and working within an appropriate clinical governance framework
- managing time and resources effectively
- being able to self-monitor and seek appropriate advice and support to maintain their own physical and mental health v demonstrating emotional resilience
- demonstrating situational awareness v reflecting on their personal behaviour and its impact on others
- demonstrating awareness of their own behaviour, particularly where this might put patients or others at risk.

(GMC, 2017: 8)

Since its inception in 2012, the Jubilee Centre for Character and Virtues based at the University of Birmingham has conducted numerous studies that have sought the views, perceptions and explanations of professionals themselves in order to interrogate and explore the ethical dimensions of professions in England, each led by the Centre's Director, Professor James Arthur. In this book, we draw on data from one of these studies – *Virtuous Medical Practice* – to present and analyse how doctors at three stages of their careers – (first year) Undergraduate Students, Graduating Students, and Experienced Doctors (we explain each of these categories below) – understand the moral dimensions of their work. While we add some additional analysis to the findings, including reporting additional qualitative data from the study and entering into conversation with relevant research literature published since the study, this book draws extensively on the original research report produced by the projects: *Virtuous Medical Practice* (Arthur et al., 2015a). The Centre's work on the ethical dimensions of medical practice as a profession has also been detailed in various articles and books published by Centre members on medical practice itself (see for example, Kristjánsson, 2015a) and on the professions more widely (for example, Arthur et al., 2015b, 2017a, 2018b, 2019b; Harrison and Khatoon, 2017; Kristjánsson et al., 2017a, 2017b).

The aim of this introductory chapter is two-fold. First, we provide summary details of the main project drawn upon in our analysis. For reasons of space and concision, we present a summary of the main aims, research questions and methods for each of these projects. The detailed aims, research questions and methods of each of these project can be found on the Jubilee Centre's website.[1] Second, we set out the structure of the book, including the focus and broad content of each of the chapters that follow.

The project

The *Virtuous Medical Practice* project was a two-year study, in Great Britain, involving first-year undergraduate medical students (referred to throughout as *Undergraduate Students*), students who had recently graduated from their course (referred to throughout as *Graduating Students*) and doctors with at least five years of experience (referred to throughout as *Experienced Doctors*). The overarching aim of the *Virtuous Medical Practice* project was to identify which personal virtues medical students and experienced doctors understood themselves as holding and to investigate how these could influence their professional lives. Specifically, the study examined how an understanding of the virtues influenced doctors' moral thinking and possible conduct, and how the environment in which doctors train and work can influence them in becoming good doctors.

The main research questions that guided the project were:

- Which virtues and values are held by members of the medical profession in the UK?
- How do doctors develop these virtues and values?
- How do virtues and values shape medical practice?
- How do these virtues and values relate to the expectations of the medical regulatory bodies?
- What are the implications of virtue-based medical ethics for ethics education in medicine?
- How can virtues and values be developed through doctors' initial training and continuing education?

The project's research design incorporated self-reporting measures of personal and professional character, as well as ethical dilemmas and extensive interviews with doctors at different stages of their careers and medical educators. The project comprised a mixed-methods, cross-sectional design. As explained in the project's final report (Arthur et al., 2015a), this design enabled the project team to examine: (1) what medical students and doctors *said* about character and medicine; (2) how considerations to do with character influence medical students' and doctor's thinking about *moral dilemmas* in medicine; and (3) the *contextual* factors that may shape and influence medical students' and doctors' character.

The project collected quantitative data through a *survey* and qualitative data through *semi-structured interviews*. The interviews enabled the project team to develop a better understanding of the conditions under which virtue can be enacted and how better to create circumstances conducive to virtue, both within the workplace and without. The survey[2] consisted of five sections (four for starting undergraduates), surveying:

1   **Respondents' views on their own character.** This comprised a list of 24 character strengths, derived from the *Values in Action Inventory of Strengths* (VIA-IS) (Peterson and Seligman, 2004) from which respondents were asked to identify the six which 'best describe the sort of person you are'.

2   **Respondents' responses to a set of moral dilemmas in their profession.** This comprised six situational judgement tests (Patterson and Ashworth, 2011; Lievens and Patterson, 2011) designed by a panel of experts (n = 15) in medical education who adapted well-known dilemmas from the literature and designed a wholly new set of answer responses specifically for this study.[3] Dilemmas were used as they (a) promise to offer a credible way to gain an insight into moral functioning and development, and (b) can ideally be designed so as to activate more than simply moral reasoning skills (Kristjánsson, 2015, chap. 3). Nevertheless, responses to dilemmas serve as an indication, rather than guarantee, of action or understanding of moral sensitivity in a real, particular situation. They do not, in and by themselves, *measure* virtue, nor do any such definitive measures exist elsewhere, but when combined with data from interviews and self-reports, they may contribute to an overall understanding of virtue in professional practice.

3   **Respondents' views on the character of the 'ideal' professional in their profession.** This comprised the list of the 24 VIA-IS character strengths presented again, with participants being asked to 'choose the six which you think best describe a good doctor'.

4   **Respondents' views regarding their work or study environment.** This section adapted questions from a Europe-wide workplace survey (The Eurofund Working Conditions Survey, 2012) with additional questions on ethical issues in the workplace.

5   **A set of demographic questions.**

Data were collected using an e-survey, the data from which was transferred to SPSS version 21, checked, cleaned and readied for analyses. Analyses included descriptive analysis, cross-tabulation, correlation and factor analysis. Analyses were also developed to deal specifically with the results of sections 1 and 3 (respondents' views on character) and section 2 (moral dilemmas).

For the semi-structured interviews, the research team devised a themed set of questions for interviews[4] with participants in the three career stages, based around the main research questions. These included questions around:

- reasons for choice of career;
- characteristics of a good professional (i.e. doctor);
- factors that can help – or hinder – being that kind of professional;
- views on the influence of character on everyday professional practice;
- the influence of the professions' code of conduct/standards; and
- the influence of education and training in developing the strengths necessary for good professional practice.

In addition to the interviews with medical students and doctors, the study also included semi-structured interviews with medical educators, for whom a separate set of questions was devised. These interviews focused on:

- their role in educating future doctors;
- their view of a good professional in their field;
- how this has changed in the course of their career;
- how students are assessed for entry;
- whether the character strengths required change and why;
- what informs their teaching in relation to the virtues; and
- how their stage of education can be developed.

In order to ensure good geographical representation, data were gathered from participants at four sites. These sites clustered around medical schools in the south of England, the midlands, the north of England and Scotland. First-year students were surveyed on entry and final year students were surveyed shortly before graduation. Interviews were also conducted with educators at these four medical schools. Practising doctors in the four regions were recruited principally with the assistance of The Royal College of General Practitioners and the Royal College of Physicians, who agreed to email links to the survey to members in those regions.

The total number of interview and survey respondents, by career stage and gender, are presented in Tables 0.1 and 0.2:

As shown in Chart 1.1, amongst practising doctors, general practitioners were the largest group in the survey sample (GMC approved single specialities). It should be noted here that the spread of numbers across the specialities prevented comparisons being made between them.

Interview participants were chosen purposively from survey participants. An invitation to interview was based on the completion of a *willingness to*

Table 0.1 Total number of respondents by career stage

Career stage	Number of surveys completed	Number of interviews conducted
Undergraduate students	122	23
Graduate students	152	24
Established doctors	275	28
Educators	n/a	10

Table 0.2 Total number of survey respondents by career stage and gender

			Career stage		
			Undergraduate students	Graduate students	Experienced doctors
Gender	Female	%	60.7%	67.1%	51.6%
	Male	%	39.3%	32.9%	48.4%

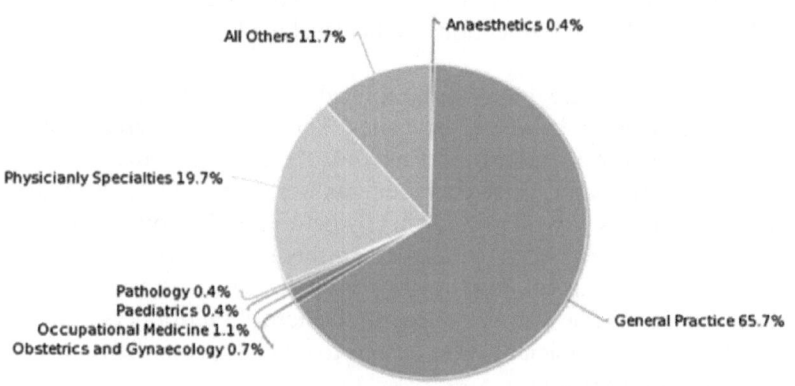

Chart 1.1 Experienced doctors by speciality.

be interviewed section on the questionnaire. Analysis of interview data was thematic, using a constant comparison (Glaser and Strauss, 1967) within a modified framework approach (Richie and Spencer, 1994). Codes were created both horizontally and vertically and then developed into categories and themes. Categories were refined and coding reviewed throughout the process for which the NVIVO software was used.

Limitations and ethical considerations

As stated in the final report of the *Virtuous Medical Practice* project (Arthur et al., 2015a), a number of limitations pertaining to the study deserve to be borne in mind. First, the study was cross-sectional. Whilst a longitudinal design would have been ideal to chart the *development* of character through medical education and practice, the time that it would have taken to track medical students from university entry to experienced practice excluded the possibility of such a design. Due to possible variation in the membership of the three cohorts studied, questions may be raised about exact comparability between the groups. A further limitation that affects all three study cohorts is response bias. More generally, surveys of character (like personality testing more generally) suffer from self-report and social desirability biases. Participation in the study was voluntary and full participation by all who were invited to respond could not be ensured. That meant that only those participants who were disposed favourably enough to the topic (whatever their views on it) responded. Consequently, the survey and interviews represented the views of a self-selected group of people and not a perfectly unbiased sample. A further limitation related specifically to the cohort of experienced professionals is that participants were contacted with the assistance of the Royal College of General Practitioners and the Royal College of Physicians which impacted on the overall profile of respondents.

The study received ethical approval from the University of Birmingham Ethics Committee. Full information regarding the study was set out in an information leaflet. As the study covered potentially sensitive topics, such as ethical dilemmas that students and doctors may have faced, all participants were asked to opt in to participation in the study. Participants' confidentiality was protected by anonymising survey responses and interview transcripts and participants were given the right to withdraw from the study up to six months after the data collection phase ended.

The structure of this book

Following this introduction, the book comprises four main chapters and a conclusion which contains a summary of the main findings, recommendations and areas for further research. Chapter 1 presents a brief review of current literature in the wider field of professional ethics. Arguing that the ethical dimension is central to what is meant by a profession, the chapter introduces the recent turn to virtues and character within literature on the professions, in particular the focus on *phronesis* (practical wisdom). In this context, the Jubilee Centre's *Building Blocks of Professional Practice* is also introduced. In Chapter 2 attention turns to the ethical nature of the medical profession. Here we contend that, as with professions more generally, the ethical forms a fundamental component of what it is that constitutes the 'good' doctor. Surveying current literature in the field, the chapter also highlights some impacts on the ethical doctor of increased marketisation and instrumentalism within healthcare systems.

In Chapters 3 and 4, data from the Virtuous Medical Practice project introduced above are presented and analysed. In Chapter 3, data are examined to consider how medical students and doctors in the study conceived character in relation to the role of the doctor and to medicine as a profession more widely. The data presented provides an initial snapshot of the motivations of the respondents to enter the medical profession and the sort of doctor (in terms of character, rather than specialism) they wished to be when embarking on their career. In addition, the chapter presents data regarding how respondents across the three career stages conceived their own personal character strengths as doctors and those character strengths they identified with the 'ideal' or 'good' doctor. In the second section, we analyse virtues in context. The chapter also examines data setting out how respondents understood the varied contextual factors that enabled and constrained their ability to practise professional virtue in their workplace settings. These responses are classified into four main headings: autonomy, involvement, support, and challenge.

In Chapter 4 we analyse responses to the series of ethical dilemmas given to the medical students and experienced doctors in the study. Based on the associations made by the expert panel, each of these three dilemmas incorporated a conflict between different virtues. In the analysis we point to the differences across and between the three career stages in terms of the chosen course of action, as well as to the reasons selected (from a pre-given list) for these choices. The chapter also considers the data across the dilemmas to report how reasons prioritised give a picture of the virtues at play (on the basis of associations between reasons and specific virtues made by the expert panel). In addition, the responses to the dilemma provided additional data regarding the role of professional codes of conduct in doctors' reasoning about the dilemmas, once again demonstrating how rules and virtues often combine in ethical decision-making. Finally, the chapters explore key themes raised in the interviews with medical educators. The book closes with *Conclusions, recommendations and further research.*

Our intention in the pages that follow is to bring together data, analysis, findings and conclusions from the *Virtuous Medical Practice* project in order to consolidate and share with new audiences what the project revealed about the ethical dimensions of medical practice and medical education, and to open up areas for further investigation that might shape the research trajectory over the coming years.

Notes

1 www.jubileecentre.ac.uk/1595/projects/virtues-in-the-professions.
2 A copy of the online survey can be found at www.jubileecentre.ac.uk/ professions.
3 For more on the design of the situational judgement tests, see www.jubilee centre.ac.uk/1595/projects/virtues-in-the-professions.
4 A copy of the interview schedule can be found at www.jubileecentre.ac.uk/ professions.

1 The professions and character

Introduction

Whether inspired by a desire to justify an occupation's status as a profession (teaching and social work, for example) or by the need to re-assert precisely what lies at the heart of a long-standing profession in the wake of public concerns about standards (medicine and law, for example), the related questions of what constitutes a profession and what constitutes professional practice have received a great deal of attention over recent years. A core concern within this literature on the professions has been to highlight and seek to understand the ethical basis of professions, whether generally or specifically. Professions are deemed inherently ethical occupations because, and more so than other occupations, they place high moral demands on the conduct of workers. Indeed, these ethical and moral demands – which include care, integrity, fairness and diligence – are often viewed as *the defining* feature of many professions, including medicine, law and teaching, reminding us that professions are ultimately concerned with *human* actions and interactions. For example, in relation to medicine, the focus of this present book, Bontemps-Hommen et al. (2019) have suggested that morality is at the heart of medicine. As Oakley and Cocking (2001) also remind us, the focus of professional work is typically the provision of goods – such as health, education and justice – that are fundamental to flourishing individuals and societies. In specific relation to medical education, Brody and Doukas (2014) talk of medicine as both a 'trust-generating profession' and as 'the application of virtue to practice' (see also Rhodes (2020) on the importance of trust). Yet, and as various professional 'scandals' over the last 20 years have evidenced, every profession and professional faces ethical challenges and dilemmas as part of their work. Indeed, the very ethical nature of the professions entails that public mistrust and criticism results when conduct falls below the standards expected (Blond et al., 2015).

DOI: 10.4324/9781003137887-2

In order to examine the ethical nature of professions and the ethical dilemmas experienced by professionals, since its inception the Jubilee Centre has undertaken a number of empirical studies examining character, virtues and the professions. Some of these studies have concentrated on the professions generally (Arthur et al., 2019a), while others have focused in on specific professions: law (Arthur et al., 2014), medical practice (Arthur et al., 2015a), education (Arthur et al., 2015b), business (Kristjánsson et al., 2017a), nursing (Kristjánsson et al., 2017b), and the British Army (Arthur et al., 2018). More recently, through the project *Practical Wisdom and Professional Practice: Integration and Intervention* the Centre has built on this research to examine particular commonalities and differences across professions and professionals (Arthur et al., 2019a).

The purpose of this first chapter is to provide an initial survey of the existing literature on the professions. The first section considers briefly what constitutes a profession in general terms, before turning to the more specific ethical dimensions of professional activity. It does so in light of the now widespread trend towards managerialism, accountability and efficiency that has been witnessed across professions in a number of countries over the last 30 years (Berwick, 2016; Montori, 2017). In the second section, attention moves to consider the value of a virtue-based account of professional ethics. In this section we draw on the Jubilee Centre's neo-Aristotelian approach to virtues and character in order to argue that professional ethics involves but also transcends reliance on rules and duties, thereby requiring professionals to act with professional wisdom and judgement.

What constitutes a profession?

While definitions of what constitutes a profession abound, certain features seem to be generally, if not universally, accepted (see, for example, Carr, 1999). These are that:

- a profession is a paid occupation;
- a profession requires formal qualifications, a high level of education and a prolonged period of training/induction;
- a professional possesses high level theoretical and practical expertise in a given discipline;
- a profession provides a public service;
- a profession is, and professionals are, held in high esteem within society;
- a professional acts with integrity, care, honesty and trust, exhibiting a level of professional autonomy and judgement;

- professional ethics is guided by a code of conduct specific to that profession.

The Australian Council of Professions,[1] which captures each of the features above, defines a 'Profession' as:

> a disciplined group of individuals who adhere to ethical standards and who hold themselves out as, and are accepted by the public as possessing special knowledge and skills in a widely recognised body of learning derived from research, education and training at a high level, and who are prepared to apply this knowledge and exercise these skills in the interest of others. It is inherent in the definition of a Profession that a code of ethics governs the activities of each Profession. Such codes require behaviour and practice beyond the personal moral obligations of an individual. They define and demand high standards of behaviour in respect to the services provided to the public and in dealing with professional colleagues. Further, these codes are enforced by the Profession and are acknowledged and accepted by the community.

In seeking to establish a 'working definition for medical educators', Cruess, Johnstone and Cruess (2004: 75) offer the following:

> An occupation whose core element is work based upon the mastery of a complex body of knowledge and skills. It is a vocation in which knowledge of some department of science or learning of the practice of an art founded upon it is used in the service of others. Its members are governed by codes of ethics and profess a commitment to competence, integrity and morality, altruism, and the promotion of the public good within their domain. These commitments form the basis of a social contract between a profession and society, which in return grants the profession a monopoly over the use of its knowledge base, the right to considerable autonomy in practice and the privilege of self-regulation. Professions and their members are accountable to those served and to society.

In the UK, various professions make clear the centrality of the 'ethical' to the nature of the profession. For example, in its Code of Ethics,[2] the British Association of Social Workers asserts that:

> Ethical awareness is fundamental to the professional practice of social workers. Their ability and commitment to act ethically is

an essential aspect of the quality of the service offered to those who engage with social workers. Respect for human rights and a commitment to promoting social justice are at the core of social work practice throughout the world.

The Law Society of England and Wales[3] makes clear that:

> The commitment to behaving ethically is at the heart of what it means to be a solicitor.
> Ethics is based on the principles of:
> * serving the interests of consumers of legal services
> * acting in the interests of justice acting with integrity and honesty according to widely recognised moral principles
> Ethics will help you respond in the right way to any moral dilemmas you might face at work.

Many more codes of conduct from other professions that similarly locate ethical conduct as fundamental to the profession could be cited. However, despite these reasonably well established and understood definitions, how best the ethical should be formulated conceptually and can be implemented practically, remains both disputed and challenging. Turning specifically to definitions of professionalism in relation to medical practice (which are examined in more detail in Chapter 2), Ong et al. (2020: 636) reflect both that rather than being static, 'professionalism is an evolving, socioculturally informed, multidimensional construct' and that 'the concept of professionalism remains poorly defined'.

Clearly, ideas about what constitutes the 'good' professional transcend simply technical abilities and encompass notions of judgement, wisdom and care. However, further questions remain about the extent to which particular cultures, discourses and practices can put pressure on how professionals, particularly those working in the public sector, can act with (or indeed without) ethics and integrity (see, for example, Furlong et al., 2017). Indeed, various studies evidence the impact (whether positive or negative) of workplace conditions on professionals' ability to exhibit ethical conduct (see, for example, Oakley and Cocking, 2001; RPS, 2011; OfSTED, 2019; Worth and Van Den Brande, 2019).

Discussions about the meaning and nature of ethical professional conduct and the effect of cultures, discourses and workplace practices typically concentrate around two particular considerations. The first is the impact, widely cited and critiqued in current literature on ethics and the professions, of the increased forms of managerialism and instrumentalism that have roundly been identified as detracting from the ethical and societal role of professionals. According to critics, the turn to manager-ialism across and within the professions has led not to a renewed form of professionalism but to a processes of de- and re-professionalisation through which the goals of general accountability (to service users and to government) and efficiency have actively worked against professional autonomy and judgement (Carr, 2011; Holbeche and Springett, 2004; Dixon-Woods et al., 2011). The second consideration is the extent to which professions, such as health, teaching and social work, have come under increased public scrutiny and accountability in the wake of various 'scandals' (Seijts et al., 2017; Arthur et al., 2019a). Over the last 25 years in England, for example, high-profile cases including the murder of Stephen Lawrence and resulting Stephen Lawrence Inquiry (known com-monly as the Macpherson Report), the murder of Victoria Climbié, the death of Peter Connelly (also known as Baby P), the Mid Staffordshire hospital crisis and the Rotherham Child Sexual Exploitation scandal have all raised serious questions about what were significant failures in professionals' ethical judgement and conduct.

In the context of managerialism, accountability, efficiency, public scrutiny and increased workplace pressures, professions and professionals need to (re)envisage the ethical nature of their work. This (re)envisaging by necessity includes paying attention to what a profes-sion aspires to be, what constitutes professional practice – whether gen-erally or specifically for that profession – and how external factors shape the standing and work of professions today (see, for example, Berwick, 2016). In the next section we start to examine these questions through a focus on a virtue-based approach to professional ethics. In doing so, we introduce key work in the field, particularly that which makes reference to the concept of professional *phronesis*.

A virtue-based approach to professional ethics

The last few decades have witnessed a groundswell of interest in virtue-based approaches to professional ethics. Though not the only variant of a virtue-ethical approach, the vast majority of this interest has drawn on Aristotelian roots, and this concerted interest in Aristotelian/neo-Aristotelian virtue has been applied across of a range of professional contexts, including accountancy (West, 2017), medicine (Pellegrino and Thomasma, 1993; Kotzee, Paton and Conroy, 2016), nursing (McKie et al., 2012), social work (Adams, 2009), and youth work (Bessant, 2009). In particular, two Aristotelian ideas have provoked significant interest among those concerned with professional ethics. The first is the idea that virtues represent 'contextually appropriate traits ... such as honesty, compassion and perseverance' that contra rules 'become habitually ingrained through deliberate and repetitive practice, predisposing practitioners to behave based on ethically sound habits' (Arthur et al., 2019a: 2). The second idea – the main focus of this section – is the concept of *phronesis*, or practical wisdom (Pellegrino and Thomasma, 1993; Gillies, 2005; Kinsella and Pitman, 2012; McKie et al., 2012). It is important to note, however, that while often cited, *phronesis* is not understood *uniformly* throughout the literature on professions (for a useful overview of *phronesis* in medical practice, see Kotzee, Paton and Conroy, 2016). Indeed, examining work on *phronesis* in professional medical ethics, Kristjánsson (2015: 299) highlights the 'considerable lack of clarity in the current discursive field on *phronesis*'.

In line with its neo-Aristotelian philosophy, the Jubilee Centre advocates the following model of the **Building Blocks of Professional Practice** (see Figure 1.1).

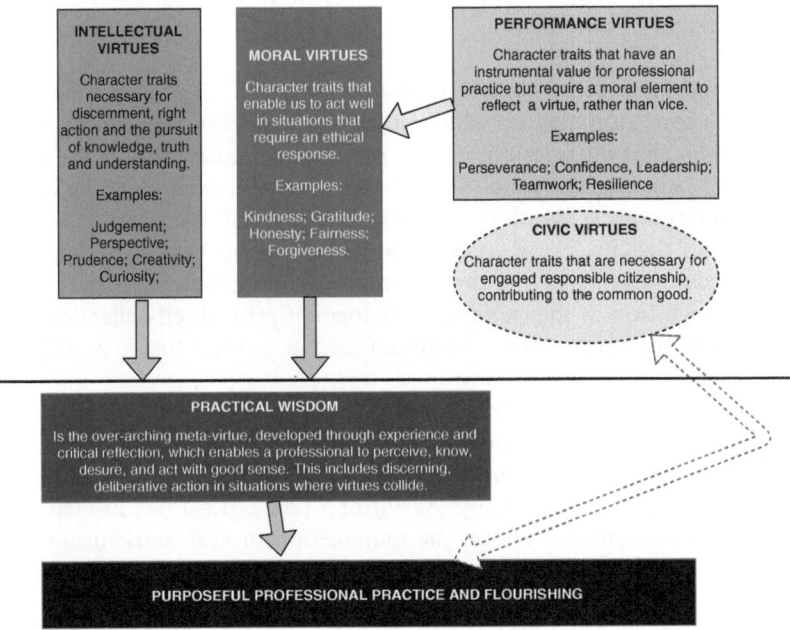

Figure 1.1 The building blocks of professional practice.
The Jubilee Centre's *A Framework for Character Education in Schools* (2017), adapted to a professional domain. The model depicts the four domains of virtue and their conceptual relationship with practical wisdom and the purposeful professional practice.

In Figure 1.1, *phronesis* – or practical wisdom – is defined as 'the over-arching meta-virtue, developed through experience and critical reflection, which enables a professional to perceive, know, desire and act with good sense. This includes discerning, deliberative action in situations where virtues collide'. In other words, professionals need a certain form of practical wisdom, or *phronesis*, which can be defined in the following way:

> To practice with *phronesis* is to act with care, diligence and open-mindedness. To practice without *phronesis* would mean acting carelessly, indecisively, and with a degree of negligence to the surrounding circumstances or possible consequences.
>
> (Arthur et al., 2019b: 5)

For some authors, it is possible and useful to identify a form of professional *phronesis* – or what Sellman (2009: 1) terms the 'professionally wise practitioner'. Sellman (2012: 116) defines the professionally wise practitioner as one who:

> continually strives to be the best practitioner she or he can be given the constraints under which practice occurs. For practitioners, this endeavour includes but is not restricted to understanding the limits of their own personal professional competencies together with a willingness to identify and work toward rectifying relevant competency deficits. These are demanding requirements that imply a deep understanding of the turbulent and dynamic nature of practice, a recognition of the value of some form of critical self-reflection, and a resolve not to allow complacency to jeopardise future practice.

Sellman makes clear that an important consideration for any virtue-based account of professional conduct and activity is to recognise the situational constraints that can act upon and constrain the ability of professionals to act ethically. As Pitman (2012: 131) has argued, and as we have suggested above, the managerialism and marketisation of public professions such as teachers, health care professionals and social workers has created a 'hostile ground for growing phronesis' (see also Dixon-Woods et al., 2011. To neglect these factors is inherently problematic. Kinsella and Pitman (2012: 8) remind us that:

> as the mechanisms of professionalization have been put in place, so too have the levels of prescription increased, thereby circumscribing the capacity of members to act autonomously in situations

that demand the exercise of judgement. The 'danger' of calling for phronesis and holding practitioners accountable for practical wisdom in contexts that may not support it, and that actively mitigate against it, is that practitioners may face a double bind, where they are blamed for a failure of agency at the personal level, when the issues may well be structural and systemic.

It is under such circumstances that moral and intellectual virtues – including the meta-virtue of *phronesis* – play a crucial role, enabling professionals to discern and deliberate about the correct course of actions given the *salient features at play* (Russell, 2009). Indeed, initial findings from a meta-analysis of professional virtues undertaken by the Jubilee Centre (Arthur et al., 2019a: 5) indicate that the '*phronetic* professional is one that is posited to endorse both moral and intellectual virtues in conjunction with one another'. These initial findings suggest 'the importance of developing a *phronetic* character profile for the enhancement of perceived professional purpose. That is, one that encompasses a value for both moral and intellectual virtue simultaneously as opposed to in isolation of one another'. Importantly, moral virtues may be crucial for developing a sense of purpose that extends beyond the self to the community in which one works', but 'it is only when a moral compass is synergised with a valuation of the intellectual virtues, that professionals are likely to experience the greatest possible sense of professional purpose' (Arthur et al., 2019a: 16). In other words, moral and intellectual values work together to guide right action and a deeper sense of professional worth.

Codes of conduct and the limitations of rule

A core feature of professional occupations, then, is the ability to handle the ethical dilemmas and challenges faced within the workplace. Professional work is such that, given the complexity of their work and challenges involved in delineating an ethically appropriate course of action, the professional cannot simply follow given guidelines or codes – particularly when ethical requirements conflict (for example, when loyalty conflicts with honesty). So too, and given the complex nature and scope of professional activity, the professional must draw on a range of salient information – theories, practices, prevalent codes, relationships involved, potential outcomes – to discern the right course of action for the right reasons (see, for example, Fish and de Cossart, 2013). In certain circumstances, the complexity and challenges of their occupation may place professionals in situations where their actions may be both morally right and yet run counter to the requirements set out by government and related agencies (Moore, 2015). As Carr (1999: 35) contends, 'responsible professional decisions must depend ultimately on the quality of *personal* deliberation and reflection'.

This is not to suggest, however, that the sort of practical wisdom needed for professional *phronesis* can be completely separated from the principles and rules that often characterise professional codes of conduct (Pellegrino and Thomasma, 1993). Having a clearly stated set of principles and rules brings a number of benefits in terms of educating new entrants to the profession, guiding professional conduct and providing those external to the profession (patients, clients, parents, pupils etc.) with some understanding of what can be expected of the profession concerned. However, rules and codes of conduct can only help the professional so far and are insufficient for true ethical practice if they are not accompanied, interpreted and balanced by intellectual and moral character. In simple terms, where codes of conduct are too rigid, cultures of conformity can undermine professional autonomy and judgement; where codes of conduct are overly ambiguous they offer professionals little by way of structure and guidance to act as a basis for their deliberations and choices.

Rules, then, may well form part of characterising ethical professional practice but in and of themselves they are an insufficient basis for true ethical practice if they are not accompanied, interpreted and balanced by intellectual and moral character. American psychologist Barry Schwartz has spoken about the ways in which the dominance of external controls, such as rules and incentives, can actively *undermine* wisdom and judgement. According to Schwartz (2009):

> rules and incentives may make things better in the short run, but they create a downward spiral that makes them worse in the long run. Moral skill is chipped away by an over-reliance on rules that deprives us of the opportunity to improvise and learn from our improvisations. And moral will is undermined by an incessant appeal to incentives that destroy our desire to do the right thing. And without intending it, by appealing to rules and incentives, we are engaging in a war on wisdom.

Importantly for the focus of this book, Schwartz (2011) has also argued that the dominance of rules and incentives does not only limit professional wisdom but also serves to undermine professional motivation. He argues that:

the problem with relying on rules and incentives is that they demoralize professional activity, and they demoralize professional activity in two senses. First, they demoralize the people who are engaged in the activity. Judge Forer quits, and Ms. Dewey is completely disheartened. And second, they demoralize the activity itself. The very practice is demoralized, and the practitioners are demoralized. It creates people – when you manipulate incentives to get people to do the right thing – it creates people who are addicted to incentives. That is to say, it creates people who only do things for incentives.

The *phronetic* professional, then, is not guided solely by duty to codes external to their own intellect and morals or by externally driven incentives, but rather conceives and applies their professional responsibilities by using their professional wisdom. This includes understanding codes of conduct, but not conceiving these as the sole arbiter when dilemmas arise. As the author C. S. Lewis (1985: 100; cited in Bohlin, 2005: 20) eloquently wrote in his *Letters to Children*:

A prefect man would never act from a sense of duty; he'd always want the right thing more than the wrong one. Duty is only a substitute for love (of God and other people), like a crutch, which is the substitute for a leg. Most of us need the crutch at times; but of course its idiotic to use the crutch when our legs (our own loves, tastes, habits etc) can do the journey on their own.

Lewis' words remind us that sound professional conduct has an internal motivation and meaning – and that is, it must come from the heart. It is for precisely this reason that many, if not all, professions are understood as vocations rather than simply occupations.

Focusing on the sorts of capacities frequently associated with professional *phronesis*, which include sensitivity, discernment, deliberation and reflection, signifies that the codification of professional conduct into a set of rules cannot be disentangled from the critical judgement of the professional. Indeed, the critical judgement of the professional is crucial if those rules are to be applied in practice, and in a way that juggles the demands of the specific situation at hand (including where stated rules may be in conflict). Whether one subscribes to an Aristotelian notion of *phronesis* that separates ethical from technical practice or from a MacIntyrean approach that understands technical practice to have an ethical dimension, it remains that the ethical is core to professional practice (Cooke and Carr, 2014; Kristjánsson, 2015b; Kotzee, Paton and Conroy, 2016).

Conclusion

In this chapter we have surveyed existing literature on the ethical dimensions of professions. As we have intimated in the chapter, it is not a question of *whether* professions such as medicine, law, nursing, social work and teaching involve an ethical dimension but rather how this dimension is and should be conceived and enacted by these professions. While general approaches to professional ethics act as a significant starting point in responding to these latter questions, the nature, demands and realities of professional ethics are necessarily moderated by the particular profession at hand. In other words, while we might approach the general ethical dimensions of professions from a given framework (in the case of the Jubilee Centre, a broadly neo-Aristotelian one), it is also necessary to appreciate that the precise ethical demands that act upon doctors, nurses, lawyers, teachers and so on are likely to be framed and expressed in ways particular to those individuals professions. With this in mind, the next chapter focuses more specifically on ethics and medical practice.

Notes

1   www.professions.com.au/about-us/what-is-a-professional.
2   www.basw.co.uk/about-basw/code-ethics.
3   www.lawsociety.org.uk/support-services/ethics/

2   Ethics and medical practice

Introduction

Broad definitions of professionalism relating to medical practice include the idea that medical practice is a *trust generating promise* (Brody and Doukas, 2014) and that questions of professionalism are fundamentally concerned with the *morality of medicine* (Bontemps-Hommen, Baart and Vosman, 2019). Inherent in the notion of medical practice as a profession is that doctors are faced with complex, difficult decisions in which they have to decide what they *could* and *should* do amongst various options. Whether they be end-of-life decisions or the subject of whether to issue a sick note, the choices and decisions facing doctors require not only medical expertise, but moral reflection and judgement. Moreover, and as Oakley and Cocking (2001: 74) explain:

> a good profession, on [a] virtue ethics approach, is one which involves a commitment to a key human good, a good which plays a crucial role in enabling us to live a humanly flourishing life ... if (as many suggest) it is appropriate to take serving health as the central goal of medicine, then given the importance of health for human flourishing, medicine would clearly count as a good profession on this approach.

Understood in these terms, illness dictates a vulnerability that is entrusted to highly trained clinician – clinicians that should be worthy of the trust vested in them by patients and, indeed, by the public more generally.

It should be recognised, too, that the ethics of everyday decisions are just as important in the life of a clinician as those decisions that relate to either life-changing or life-ending medical care. Central to clinical practice is the extent to which decisions bring together competing

DOI: 10.4324/9781003137887-3

perspectives – and indeed virtues. Relevant here, for example, is that medical consultations involve an interplay of the patient's stance and desires, the clinician's perspective and judgement, and the wider dictates of the profession and society. In each of these, moral perspectives and principles are involved. In practice, the patient and the doctor oscillate between perceiving the body as an object and a subject (Heath, 2015). Biomedical science helps address the body as an object, addressing disease and dysfunction as a mechanical problem that can be fixed. The more complicated aspect of medicine is the patient as a subject; that is their illness narrative. Here, patients may place subjective, and ultimately moral, projections in their stories – stories that are then subjectively interpreted by the clinician who in turn projects their own moral perspective on the story.

This chapter is interested in the ethical dimensions of medical practice and, more specifically, with the centrality of ethics for what it means to be a 'good' doctor. Offering a narrative review (we do not claim this to be a comprehensive review given the space possible) of existing literature in the field, the chapter positions the moral dimensions of medical practice and medical education within the wider field of virtue ethics, describing the limitations of rules-based ethics in this area. Having done so, it then considers the importance of *phronesis* – or practical wisdom – for medical practice. The chapter is divided into three main sections. In the first, and building on the wider review in the last chapter, we make some initial comments about medical practice as a profession. In the second section, we examine the importance of doctors' character taking account of current pressures placed upon medical practice within increasingly marketised healthcare systems. In the final section we focus on the character of doctors and, more specifically, on the importance of *phronesis* – or practical/professional wisdom.

Medical practice as a profession

Medicine is a classical profession. One of the three original 'liberal professions', along with the priesthood and the law, nothing sets medicine apart from other spheres of work as much as the ethical relationship between the doctor and their patients. Doing justice to this relationship over a lifetime of practice arguably demands not only adherence to an ethical code that governs the profession, but also the self-awareness and desire to nurture various dispositions – indeed virtues – such as compassion, care, honesty curiosity, creativity, courage, teamwork, humour and a sense of fairness. In short, being a doctor calls for the continuous development of good professional character. If we consider, for example, the expectations of doctors found within the General Medical Council's *Good Medical Practice* (2019: 4; emphasis added) guidelines the importance of character is clear, if not necessarily fully developed. The guidelines state, for example, that

> Good doctors make the care of their patients their first concern: they are competent, keep their knowledge and skills up to date, establish and maintain *good relationships* with patients and colleagues, are *honest* and *trustworthy*, and act with *integrity* and within the law.

The guidelines also state that good doctors 'work in *partnership with patients* and respect their rights to privacy and dignity', and that doctors 'must use [their] *judgement* in applying the principles to the various situations [they] will face as a doctor'.

Of course, while the character and judgement of doctors is fundamental to their work and relationships with patients, medical practice today takes place within specific regulatory, institutional, political, and economic frameworks. Over at least the last three decades (and as we survey in this chapter) a number of studies across a range of contexts have suggested a deep and growing interest in the professional ethics of medicine. A relatively common and persistent theme in this literature is the impact of healthcare reforms on the environments in which doctors work. With specific regard to the United Kingdom, for example, it is clear both that the healthcare needs of the UK's population and the environments in which care is delivered are changing rapidly. Moreover, political devolution is leading to growing differences in the way healthcare is organised and delivered in the four countries of the UK. This ongoing healthcare reform, especially major structural change in England, has raised further uncertainty about the future shape of healthcare and its capacity to meet future demand. The nature of doctors' work is, then, ever-evolving in large part due to the complex and changing contexts in which it occurs (Jha et al., 2006, 2007; Christmas and Millward, 2011). Given regular changes in the types, effectiveness and cost of medical treatment as well as shifting demographic and societal changes, there is consistent pressure on the medical profession to be able to manage complex and fluid contextual factors in ways that combine economic, moral and other considerations. More recently, the Covid-19 global pandemic has added further change and complexity. While the long-term impacts are not yet known for certain, in the short term, the pandemic has led to significant restrictions on the scope of routine medical and surgical work in hospitals, while general practice surgeries have moved to conducting the majority of appointments remotely. This remote work – while potentially more immediately efficient – often denies clinicians and their patients close, in-person contact, perhaps leading to less joyful and more transactional consultations. Such concerns about online consultations were raised before the pandemic (BBC, 2017), and have been raised since with the chair of the Royal College of General Practitioners stating that online calls felt like 'working in a call centre', meaning that GPs could not pick up on 'soft cues' central to diagnoses (Campbell, 2021).

It should also be noted that doctors' work – including the ethical dimensions of this work – occurs under ever greater scrutiny and accountability. Indeed, the impact of market-led reforms medical practice, on healthcare more generally, and on wider public services are well-attested. In this context, and similarly to other public service professionals such as nurses and teachers, a core task facing doctors is to mediate the negative impacts of marketisation. In other words, doctors are involved in a continual process of working within the constraints and demands while trying to enact their professionalism. However, and as Berwick (2016: 1329) states, 'when the ethos of professionalism clashes with the ethos of markets and accountability immense resources get diverted from the crucial and difficult enterprise of creating care'. Similarly, in their research on emergency medicine and emergency physicians, Larkin et al. (2009: 52) speak of how marketisation subverts the true nature of the profession, asserting:

> that the telos of an EP [emergency physician] is not merely to work within the rules, but also to be a moral professional who cares for and about patients. This notion transcends corporate and contractual requirements. While the recognition of virtue does not prevent the sound application of business principles to the practice and management of medicine, it does prevent finances from becoming the solitary driving force.
>
> (Larkin et al., 2009: 52)

Oftentimes, the impact of policies may be unintended – or at least have conflicting affects. An illustrative case in point is the (real and/or perceived) impact of the European Working Time Directive on the education and training of junior doctors in England. While on one hand the Directive strived to protect junior doctors (and indeed their patients) from excessive time spent on-call at the same time, as Rodriguez-Jareño et al (2014: 1) noted, the Directive 'has been associated with concerns about the provision of health services including continuity of care, lower staffing levels, introduction of shift working, a reduction in training time and the adequate supervision of junior doctors'.

A particular educational challenge of the current context, then, is to adapt to a world of higher expectations and wider responsibilities where, at the same time and more than ever, doctors will be expected to develop and exercise professional virtues in order to work with and lead multi-disciplinary teams, deal with uncertainty, and to understand the various systems in which they work. In other words, doctors, and indeed the medical professions more widely, have to aspire to excellence within highly pressurised systems with competing agendas in which burnout, self-sacrifice, and other concerns are both evident and persistent and in which attempts to reduce the burden on doctors (i.e. working patterns, the use of online technologies etc.) have notable downsides for their practice. In such contexts the flourishing of medical professionals, patients, other stakeholders and, indeed, of healthcare systems and wider societies are constrained.

In light of these latter comments, Berwick's (2016) casting of 'three eras' of healthcare provides an interesting account. According to Berwick, Era 1 represents the foundations of the medical profession and is characterised by beneficence and self-regulation. Era 2, which Berwick suggests is found in contemporary healthcare environments, is characterised by measurement and systems of 'rewards and punishment'. These two eras noted, Berwick advances nine changes needed to advance a third era – a moral era – typified by transparency, greater freedoms from scrutiny and increased civility. Crucially, within these changes Berwick (2016: 1330; see also Hannah, 2014) includes the need to 'hear the voices of the people served', arguing that:

> The more patients and families become empowered, shaping their care, the better that care becomes, and the lower the costs. Clinicians, and those who train them, should learn how to ask less, 'What is the matter with you?' and more, 'What matters to you?' 'Coproduction,' 'co-design,' and 'person-centered care' are among the new watchwords, and professionals, and those who train them, should master those ideas and embrace the transfer of control over people's lives to the people. That includes paying special attention to the needs of the poor, the disadvantaged, and the marginalized, and firmly defending health care as a universal human right.

It is important to note here, too, that medical education and training are also being provided in this changing environment, with UK curricular reforms having been introduced in medical schools in order to keep pace with internal and external changes to the medical profession. However, while the education, training and career paths of junior doctors may have changed in some important regards, some studies have suggested a predominance of positivist bioscience in most undergraduate medical curricular, with much less attention paid to the intricacies and complexities of the moral dimensions of medical practice (see, for example, Hilton and Southgate, 2007). In this context, medical students may struggle with the volume of assessed factual content, trying to grasp how to prioritise workload and manage other more expedient concerns rather than focusing on the moral essence of the profession. There is, for instance, some research to show that medical students' capacity for moral reasoning at best remains stagnant through medical school; some studies show a decline (Serodio, Kopelman and Bataglia, 2016).

Why doctors' character matters

Broadly and generally, the medical profession itself, and doctors more specifically, are held in high esteem. Polls of public trust in the professions regularly find that doctors are the professionals most trusted by the British public; an Ipsos MORI poll in 2011, for example found that 88 per cent, nearly nine out of ten adults in the UK trust doctors to tell the truth (Ipsos MORI, 2011). An Ipsos MORI poll in 2017 found that while nurses were the most trusted profession – 94 per cent of respondents trusted they would tell the truth – doctors were trusted to tell the truth by 91 per cent of respondents (Ipsis MORI, 2017). A 2015 analysis by the Kings Fund (Charles, 2015) using data from the British Social Attitudes Survey found that between 2002 and 2014 'public trust in doctors remained broadly unchanged'. In addition, those with more recent contact with NHS services (i.e. in the previous 12 months) expressed greater levels of trust in doctors than those who had not.

However, some studies have suggested that public trust in the medical profession may be declining across a range of countries (see, for example, Huang et al., 2018; Blendon et al., 2014). While a number of factors influencing declining and/or differential levels of trust in the medical profession have been advanced, two seem particularly relevant. The first explanation, which we have touched upon already, is the commodification and commercialisation of healthcare and healthcare systems. More precisely, in those countries where healthcare and healthcare systems are more commodified and commercialised (e.g. greater privatisation; a focus on market-led access to and allocation of treatments, and so on) levels of public trust are reduced. Conversely, some evidence seems to suggest levels of increased trust in regions aspiring to 'humanising healthcare' (Hannah, 2014).

A second factor influencing falling levels of trust (at times better framed in terms of the *changing* nature of trust) is that high-profile scandal and transgressional behaviour by doctors and other healthcare professionals may be re-shaping public perceptions. Investigations of high-profile cases in the UK, such as the unacceptably high death-rate of babies undergoing heart surgery at the Bristol Royal Infirmary and the organ retention scandal at Alder Hey Children's Hospital, have highlighted a number of issues. These issues include concerns over not only clinical competency, but also the ethical behaviour of some doctors and the effectiveness of monitoring by hospital authorities (Department of Health, 2001; Hall, 2001). More recently, the report on the Mid-Staffordshire NHS hospital scandal, chaired by Sir Robert Francis QC, highlighted the interplay between numerous factors. The Report identified several connected issues, including aspects of the culture of the Trust, standards and methods of compliance, poor communication, and the effects of repeated reorganisation of the Trust. Indeed, the explanations of the Trust's failings considered within the report detail a picture in which systemic and cultural weaknesses impeded on and constrained the character of professionals and other healthcare workers. The report states, for example, that patients were treated with 'callous indifference' (Great Britain. Parliament. House of Commons, 2013: 13). Francis is also reported to have stated that 'there was a lack of care, compassion, humanity and leadership' at the Trust (*The Independent*, 7 February 2013).

These two factors are not, of course, the only ones that are at play in the ongoing and fluid nature of trust between medical professionals, their patients and the wider public. The thoughts of Tallis (2006), who suggests that problems within the medical profession will always attract more media attention than gradual improvements to good practice, still resonate. In addition, Tallis identified three developments that had altered the standing of the medicine as a profession, namely: advances in technology that have enabled medical information to be more widely available to patients, less deference from patients and a greater inclination to challenge medical expertise, and an intensification in levels of 'consumerism' that have increased patient expectations placed upon doctors (Tallis, 2006: 7). As a result, doctors do not only need to be experts at diagnoses and delineating the appropriate course of action, but in communicating their judgements and in managing the expectations of patients. The contemporary emphasis on shared decision-making between doctor and patient means that an 'old model' of medical professionalism 'characterised by paternalism, emotional disengagement and establishing certainty' has been replaced by an emphasis on 'patient-centeredness and collaboration' (Borgstrom, Cohn and Barcley, 2010: 1330). This move towards collaboration extends the moral and intellectual demands on doctors, requiring them to be sensitive to and express the professional virtues of trustworthiness, empathy, openness, and compassion amongst others in order to cultivate a shared understanding of medical practice and interventions. This shared understanding represents a fusion of evidence-based medicine, shared decision making and patient-centred medicine (Lehman, 2017).

A further point is relevant here. Given the widespread view that patients' expectations of doctors and wider healthcare provisions are rising, it is useful to draw a distinction between *interactional, relationship based care* and *transactional care*. According to Iles, Sweeney and Vaughan Smith (2009: 3), while the latter focuses on 'efficiency', 'effectiveness', 'predetermined protocols' and 'reflection on facts and figures', the former focuses on the 'quality of the moment', 'emergent creativity', and 'reflection on feelings and ethics'. Writing in the *BMJ* last year, Helen Salisbury (2020: 1), a General Practitioner, suggests that transactional care is suggestive that 'we're "good" doctors if we can tick the boxes in the Quality and Outcomes Framework, follow guidelines, and keep within our prescribing budgets'. In contrast, relational care recognises that 'relationships and trust develop over time', while 'continuity of care brings a reduction in medical activity – fewer investigations performed, fewer medicines prescribed and referrals made'. The latter approach is not, of course, necessarily straightforward or easy, requiring doctors to show empathy and to open themselves up to patient–physician interaction to a great degree (Ruzycki, Traboulsi and Stanley-Bhanji, 2018).

Doctors of character

In the field of medical ethics, the concept of moral character or 'virtue' has experienced a revival over the last three decades. A virtue is a morally evaluable character trait of a person (such as honesty or courage), and we can include within such traits essential intellectual qualities, or virtues, such as open-mindedness, intellectual humility and curiosity. Interest in virtue and medical practice has, on this basis, concentrated largely on the moral and intellectual character of medical practitioners. The revival in interest in virtue ethics, character and medical practice can be traced to the early 1990s and the work of authors such as Pellegrino and Thomasma (1993) who drew on the wider revival in virtue ethics within moral philosophy to offer analysis of the virtues of the good, professional doctor (Arthur et al., 2015a). To an important extent this interest in virtue ethics and the character of doctors was a response to principle- or rule-based approaches to medical ethics in which the work of doctors was delimited and informed by certain guiding principles to which medical professionals adhere. The renewed focus on character emphasised both the judgement of the medical professional and, as mentioned above, a more interactional conception of doctor–patient relationship within which decision-making is both a moral endeavour and includes a focus on the flourishing (*eudaimonia*) of the patient (Toon, 2014).

Within the literature on the virtues of medical practice, particular virtues or character strengths have been cited as commensurate with the 'good' doctor. Alongside trustworthiness, qualities such as compassion, empathy, openness, and respect for the patient have been emphasised as central to and for ethical practice and, importantly, doctor–patient relationships (Borgstrom, Cohn and Barclay, 2010). According to McDougall (2013: 23–24):

> The virtuous doctor is seen as compassionate and benevolent, engaging with patients sensitively and caringly. The good doctor is also posited as truthful, but in a way shaped by his or her compassion; the medical virtue of truthfulness is not just brutal honesty. The virtuous doctor is just, allocating resources including his or her own skills on ethical grounds. Facing the combination of medical complexity, human mortality, and vast technological possibilities, the virtuous doctor is appropriately humble about the possibility that treatment may fail. Altruism is presented as a further character trait of the good doctor. He or she is to some degree self-sacrificing, putting patients' needs first.

The growing support for a virtue-based approach to medical ethics (Coulehan, 2005; Bryan and Babelay, 2009; Toon, 2014) has included important discussions about the purpose and content of the education of medical professionals, not least about whether medical ethics should concentrate on developing and understanding of key principles/codes of ethical conduct (including reasoning about those principles/codes) or, in addition, on the development and expression of doctors' character. Eckles et al. (2005: 1145) has referred to this as the 'skill/virtue' dichotomy. The question is whether the essential purpose of medical ethics is to promote skills in reasoning and arguing about the principles of good medical practice, or whether it should aim, instead, to influence the character of real doctors in line with the goals of medicine towards flourishing. As stated in the report on which this book is based (Arthur et al., 2015a: 9):

> advocates of rule-based approaches stress the advantages of systematising thinking about medical ethics by seeing all problems of medical ethics in terms of a small number of principles (such as the famous four principles of medical ethics of Beauchamp and Childress (1979) – beneficence, non-maleficence, justice and autonomy). Advocates of virtue approaches, on the other hand, stress the abstract nature of these principles and hold that, without a good deal of information about context, the four principles themselves do not provide a road-map to making ethical decisions in medicine.

While there is not scope in this chapter to pay full attention to the intricacies of this debate, it is important to reiterate a contention offered in the previous chapter, namely that any meaningful approach to professional ethics must account for principles while not viewing such principles as the sole basis or guide for moral professionals (in this sense, the important emphasis should be not be on a direct *choice* between principles and character, but on how character moves beyond principles in an informed way and how medical professionals work with and between principles and their character). As Pellegrino and Thomasma (1993: 19) argued cogently, principles are 'too abstract [and] that their use in moral judgments is too formularised and far removed from the concrete human particulars of moral choice'. Moreover, principles are often of less help in guiding conduct and practice in complex professional contexts, such as when principals conflicts.

A core benefit of virtue approaches to medical ethics is that they seek to provide an account of *good judgement* as an educable virtue. Kaldjian (2010), for example, identifies strong similarities between wise ethical judgement in medicine and 'clinical judgement', both of which 'requires repetitive and supervised practice over years of training so that trainees can learn a skill that comes by experience ...' (Kaldjian, 2010: 560–561). This educational experience in developing good judgement requires a reflective capacity towards knowing and doing good, which stands in comparison to much of 'modern medicine' that 'has become steeped in the tradition of rules, laws, scientific principles, and utilitarian practice guidelines' (Larkin et al., 2009: 52). As Pellegrino (1995: 264) remarked in his seminal text on a virtue-based approach to the ethics of health professions, the rise of principle-based ethics in the mid-to-late twentieth century:

> appealed to health professionals as being more definitive than virtue because of its concreteness and applicability to clinical decisions. Second, socio-political change toward participatory democracy, greater public education, distrust of authority, and the character failings of some physicians focused public attention on autonomy-based, contractual relationships rather than trust-based, covenantal ones. Third, and importantly, the religious and philosophical consensus that undergirded professional ethics, at least in the West, was challenged and weakened.

A much noted – and critiqued – implication of a principle-based rather than character-based approach to the ethics of medical practice is that codes of conduct typically set out a *minimum* standard of ethical practice and can encourage an attitude of *compliance*. In contrast, and as Barilan and Brusa (2012: 5) suggest, an understanding of the moral dimensions of the medical profession rooted in virtue ethics is 'excellence-oriented'. This view, as we considered in Chapter 1 in relation to professions more generally, understands that

> familiarity or even an ability to recite the entire ethical code and ethical guidelines without missing a punctuation mark does not guarantee ethical conduct and professionalism. Internalisation of the profession's moral edict has to take place before it can manifest as attitudes and behaviour.
>
> (Campbell and Chin, 2011: 1–2)

To rehearse from earlier in this book, this view does not negate the value of codes of ethics. Rather it sees these as performing a necessary but not sufficient role in guiding the conduct and decisions of doctors:

> Ordinary situations that require clarification of the role (expectations of a professional in given situations) and strength of will (e.g. refusing a kickback) appear to benefit most from explicit codes. On the other hand, extraordinary situations call upon virtuous persons to be guided mainly by their internal moral resources and to take courageous and even controversial actions (e.g. disconnecting a respirator, resisting unjust instructions by superiors and exercising conscientious refusal). As clinical medicine often deals with the vulnerable and unusual in the human condition, over-codification

may constrain virtuous behaviors in situations that appear to resist universalization and closure. As wisdom and expertise are about coping with the unexpected, and unknown with flexibility and creativity codes that anticipate specific scenarios are of little help in the face of many clinical problems.

(Barilan and Brusa, 2012: 5)

Turning to medical education, cultivating good medical professionals cannot be narrowly focused on knowledge and adherence to a given code of conduct or principles, nor even with wise reasoning about such principles (Goldie, 2012). Rather, the ethical development of doctors must also be concerned with recognising and nurturing the character of the good doctor. It is about knowing what the goals of medicine are and using one's knowledge and character to contextualise every patient interaction towards that goal. (For a critique of this view see, for example, Veatch, 2006). It is important to remember here too (and we return to this point in later chapters) that interest in character and a humanitarian approach to medical practice play an important role in motivating those entering the medical profession. In addition, there is evidence to show that moral reasoning skills decline as students progress through medical school (Serodio, Kopelman and Bataglia, 2016). A vital question, therefore, remains how medical education cultivates, sustains and – perhaps at times inhibits – the moral motivations, altruism and enthusiasm of new entrants to the profession.

Central to this latter question lies the cultivation of *phronesis*, the integrative, meta-virtue which enables the clinician to perceive, know, desire and act with good sense (there is not scope here to enter the full terrain of conceptual contestation and unambiguity still at play in regard to the various usages of *phronesis* in medical literature, not least with regard to the interplay between technical and moral aspects of doctors' work. For a detailed consideration see Kristjánsson, 2015). Broadly speaking, though by no means applicable to all invocations of the concept in medicine, *phronesis* – also phrased as *professional wisdom* or *prudence* – enables the clinician to grasp the morally salient features of the situation and factor these into their clinical decisions alongside many other variables and conflicts, avoiding excess and deficiency (for an interesting discussion of character failings in surgeons from a character perspective, see Elledge and Jones, 2020). There has been great interest not only in the importance of *phronesis* for medical practice, but in how it can be developed in medical students (Pellegrino and Thomasma, 1993; Hilton and Slotnick, 2005; Kinghorn, 2010; Kazzam, 2010; Kladjian, 2010; Kotzee, Paton and Conroy, 2016; Paton and Kotzee, 2019; Cardenas,

2020). Crucially, it is this professional wisdom that enables doctors to respond to the various contextual features of a given situation. Indeed, for advocates of virtue-based approaches to ethical medical practice, this contextual adaptability is of fundamental importance. According to Dowie (2000: 241) 'when a clinical decision has to be made in a given situation, phronesis brings reflection to bear upon the appropriate action to take, depending on the concrete circumstances'. Pellegrino (1995: 270) speaks of the central role of prudence, suggesting that:

> Knowing how to unscramble apparent conflicts among the virtues, understanding their relationships to one another, and selecting the means by which to approximate most closely the telos of any particular healing relationship are essential tasks for the virtue of prudence in the health professions.

Walker (2005: 1680) similarly argues that:

> Clinical encounters typically involve calls to multiple virtues – compassion, justice, courage, gentleness, or tolerance for example – and it is not uncommon for these to pull in different directions. For example, it can be difficult to know if it would be better to scold a noncompliant patient or to be empathetic. Some situations require courage more than tact, others justice more than compassion. Prudence, a meta-virtue, helps to steer the right course.

For many, and whatever the theoretical merits, the attention paid to doctors' character and decision-making in specific contexts speaks to the reality of clinical practice. As MacDougall (2013: 27) argues, for example, 'this approach better reflects the junior doctor's experience as 'an ethically complex and challenging one ... [and] captures the various moral considerations at play more comprehensively than either principlism or consequentialism'. Yet, and as was the case when the study on which this book is based was conducted, despite several other studies in recent years, it remains the case that empirical understandings of 'clinical-judgements as *phronesis* are rare' (Conroy et al., 2021; see also Paes, Leat and Stewart, 2018; Stenersen Hovdenak and Wiese, 2018).

Conclusion

A recent Editorial (2020: 126) of the *British Journal of Oral and Maxillofacial Surgery* speaks of the need for a 'paradigm shift in the ways doctors are being trained', a shift that is 'increasing being recognised'.

This move is the 'adoption of character reformation as a legitimate aim of medical education', including crucially a focus on *phronesis*. As we have suggested in this chapter, medical practice is in large part constituted by deep moral interactions and relationships between patients and doctors within complex settings. As Atul Gawande (2011: 19) wrote in his book *The Checklist Manifesto*, 'Medicine has become the art of managing extreme complexity – and a test of whether such complexity can, in fact, be humanly mastered'. Where healthcare practice and medical education is dominated by rules-based ethics, minimum standards rather than excellence of practice are prioritised in pursuit of uniformity of delivery. Such an approach lends itself to regulation, to measurement and to the management of efficiency. However, rules can be applied unreflectively and without real engagement with the moral imperative (Schultz and Carnevale, 1996), running the risk of failing to capture the heart of medical practice, alienated clinicians from altruistic goals of service to humanity (McKinley et al., 2020). As the aforementioned Editorial concluded, rather than asking which rules doctors should follow, the focus instead should be on the kind of people they are and can become. The ethical dimensions of medical education and training, therefore, should be directed to the complexities and ambiguities of medical practice, placing character at the core. To quote directly once again, 'the rewards will be free-thinking, balanced, and measured decision-makers who may flourish … in their clinical career and have a deep-seated and worthwhile happiness that nowadays eludes so many in the practice of modern medicine' (Editorial, 2020: 127).

3   Medical practitioners

Personal and ideal character strengths

Introduction

In this chapter we present, analyse and discuss empirical data drawn from the Jubilee Centre project – *Virtuous Medical Practice* (Arthur et al., 2015) – which examined how the medical students and doctors in the study conceived character in relation to the roles of the doctor and to medicine as a profession more widely. The chapter consists of two main sections. In the first, data is presented that provides an initial snapshot of the motivations of the respondents to enter the medical profession and the sort of doctor (in terms of character, rather than specialism) they wished to be when embarking on their career. In addition, the first section presents data regarding how respondents across the three career stages conceived their own personal character strengths as doctors and those character strengths they identified with the 'ideal' or 'good' doctor. In the second section, we analyse virtues in context. Here we present data setting out how respondents understood the varied contextual factors that enabled and constrained their ability to practise professional virtue in their workplace settings. These responses are classified into four main headings: autonomy, involvement, support, and challenge. By exploring these themes, we consider the key features of the workplace that influence virtuous practice.

Personal motivations and virtues

As explained in the introduction to this book, the *Virtuous Medical Practice* project sought the views of respondents at various stages of the medical careers on their own personal character strengths as well as those they equated with the 'ideal' doctor. In this section, we present respondents' views of their personal character but before doing so we present, first, analysis of data obtained through the interviews

DOI: 10.4324/9781003137887-4

with respondents regarding their motivations for entering the medical profession.

Analysis of the qualitative data suggests that respondents across the three career stages reported varied reasons behind their decision to become a doctor. For some respondents, the motivations stated were relatively pragmatic, as the following example illustrates:

> *It's a varied job and I didn't want something where I sat down at a desk all day. It's intellectually challenging and stimulating and lots of chance to interact with people.*
>
> (Graduating Student)

For many respondents, and perhaps not unsurprisingly, different forms of motivations were at play in the responses provided:

> *Everyone asks that question all the time and I don't really have an answer. I've always wanted to be a doctor and since I was about 9 I just knew. I don't have anyone in the family who's a doctor and no particular reasons except that I love science, I love people – it just seemed a logical choice. It seemed like something I wanted to do.*
>
> (Graduating Student)

Indeed, oftentimes it was this combination between a 'love of science' and 'love of people' that was at the fore of the motivations spoken about by respondents:

> *I chose medicine because I wanted a job that wasn't really centred around me and about gaining money. I wanted something that would help other people and have a significant impact on society directly and something where – that was involved with science.*
>
> (Graduating Student)

> *I suppose what I wanted to do was to be kind and to be good at it so that I was able to make good decisions and good diagnoses … like most people starting medicine I was immensely idealistic … I think I viewed it as a dedicated profession where you could use science, which I loved, for the welfare of people and humankind and maybe research and the cure of diseases and just the idea I guess of making a difference and doing something for humanity. So that was a sort of idealistic basis I think.*
>
> (Experienced Doctor)

Interestingly, however, while further attesting to the combination of a love of science and a love of people, one respondent – a Graduating Student – mentioned that the motivation of 'helping others' was not one that would necessarily go down well in certain circumstances:

It [reason for entering the profession] was definitely a combination of things. Unfortunately I mean everyone when you go for interview says 'Don't say it's to help people' but I think most people go into medicine to help people. There's definitely an aspect of really enjoying science and questioning everything, you know why does this happen and trying to be a bit of a detective with the human body but there's also an element of wanting to get people better and that's what I mean to help people. So it's kind of a combination of science and people.

(Graduating Student)

Of further note across the interviews is that while character-driven reasons were not always given in terms of motivation to become a doctor this did not mean that being an ethical professional was not at the forefront of respondents' conception of the type of doctor they were and/or wanted to become. The following two extracts, both from Graduating Students are illustrative of the more nuanced role of personal character in regard to becoming a doctor:

As I got to my third year in [my] degree I thought, well, I'm learning all of this sort of medical science without any of the clinical side of it and I really thought I'd be much more interested in the clinical side of it than the medical side, so after that, I wasn't sure if I wanted to do teaching or not, so I worked in a school for about six months, really didn't enjoy it, so then was determined to pursue a career in Medicine, so I worked as a healthcare assistant to be sure that that's what I wanted to do … I feel like I'm a good communicator and I think a lot of people who I discussed the sort of option with at the time said, you know, you'd be excellent, you're really good at talking to people and you're a very caring person.

(Graduating Student)

I think before I actually started Medicine, the reason why I wanted to do it was because, it was two-fold, one because I enjoyed Science, you know, I was always interested in how things worked and you know, physiology and the second important reason was because I wanted to actually offer help and you know, provide care to people. I wanted something where I can actually marry those two together, so that was

> *my sort of main reason ... I wanted to be a caring doctor, who was professional, you know, who met my patients' needs, you don't just treat them but also understood, you know, where they were coming from as well, why they're actually presenting in the first place.*
>
> (Graduating Student)

In these extracts we see each of the graduating students reasoning through their respective motivations for joining the profession, while also drawing links between their own character and perceptions of being a good doctor. So far as the undergraduate students were concerned, and reflecting wider academic and public discourse on healthcare professions, in the interviews compassion was often at the centre of the type of doctor the students wanted to be. For example, one respondent explained that:

> *I think also sort of personal attributes, as well. I sort of want to develop ... being compassionate, being ... having sort of integrity, honesty, so that patients can trust you. I think those are just as important as sort of the academic side of medicine.*
>
> (Undergraduate Student)

Interestingly, in speaking of the virtues they wished to exhibit as a doctor, some of the undergraduate students spoke at the same time of the existent pressures that would constrain their professionalism:

> *Definitely compassionate, I mean, I know doctors get a lot of stick about not being compassionate and, I don't know, you hear things now as a medical student and you think that's what I don't want to be like and I think by the time I've finished my course I'll realise how much hard work it is and how much time you don't have with the patient that you can't really get across how compassionate you are but that, at the moment, that's something, that's my one key focus, that's what I def- initely want to do, so.*
>
> (Undergraduate Student)

Moving now to the personal virtues reported in the survey, in the project, and mirroring the approach taken in other projects focusing on professions conducted by the Jubilee Centre, respondents were provided with a list of 24 character strengths from which to choose to describe their own personal character and that of the ideal doctor (from Peterson and Seligman's *Character Strengths and Virtues Classification,*

2004). Respondents were asked to rank the six character strengths they thought best reflected their personal character.

Across the responses, doctors and medical students evidenced a strong degree of consistency regarding the personal character strengths reported. Of the 24 strengths, five were selected by respondents across all three career stages as best reflecting their character:

- fairness;
- honesty;
- kindness;
- perseverance; and
- teamwork.

This consistency noted, one small difference that did emerge between cohorts regarding their reported personal character strengths was that graduate students reported that they possessed the strength of humour to a greater degree than first-year undergraduates (this finding is significant at the 0.05 level, $p < 0.05$). In addition, the analysis found several differences based on respondents' gender. Female respondents were more likely to report kindness as a personal strength than male respondents, while the latter were more likely to report humour as a personal strength ($p < 0.05$). Across the respondents, the three least reported personal character strengths were bravery, prudence and zest. Table 3.1 shows the percentage of choices for each character strength.[1]

Returning to the interview data, when asked about the qualities they hoped to demonstrate as a medical practitioner three largely stood out: being caring, being trustworthy and having a good relationship with patients. For some respondents, the more specific qualities, such as care and trust, were spoken of as forming the foundation for productive relationships with patients. For example, one of the undergraduate students spoke of their hope 'to be the kind of doctor that the local people would trust and feel it was easy to talk to'.

Reflecting on their intentions when joining the profession, one of the experienced doctors interviewed explained:

I think I wanted to be a caring one and someone who was with their patients rather than separate from them, if that makes sense. And I think someone who talked – you know, who talked and listened would always have been high on my list.

Table 3.1 Respondents' reported personal character strengths

Figures in %	Undergraduate students	Graduate students	Experienced doctors
Appreciation of beauty	1	2	2
Bravery	1	1	1
Creativity	3	3	2
Curiosity	7	5	5
Fairness	8	8	10
Forgiveness	3	2	2
Gratitude	3	3	2
Honesty	9	9	11
Hope	2	1	2
Humour	5	8	7
Judgement	4	3	4
Kindness	9	10	8
Leadership	5	4	5
Love	2	3	2
Love of learning	6	6	5
Modesty	4	3	3
Perseverance	8	7	6
Perspective	3	4	4
Prudence	1	1	1
Self-regulation	3	2	3
Social intelligence	2	5	4
Spirituality	2	1	3
Teamwork	6	7	7
Zest	1	1	1

A theme that emerged across the interviews with experienced doctors was that whilst formal education had prepared them to be *knowledgeable* and *competent* about and in medicine, a broader set of qualities had been learnt through experience, whether in the workplace or their wider lives. The following experienced doctor framed their experiences as involving a shift from a 'task oriented' approach to one in which spending time and getting to know patients (and the attendant qualities) came to the fore:

> *I think when you're a junior doctor, it's so sort of task orientated, what you're doing, you're running from one task to another, I don't think I, through much of my early years as a junior doctor, I thought a great deal about that. I think when I became a registrar (…) I spent more time talking to patients, partly 'cause I did more clinics, so you spend more time seeing patients, you get to know patients a little bit*

better and it's more common that you have to explain, give bad news to patients, speak to relatives, so you then start to appreciate some of the importance of empathy and valuing patients' beliefs, etc.

While the doctors with more years in the medical profession were able to discuss their actual experiences, it was notable that the views and expectations of the less experienced doctors were not dissimilar. In the interviews, the graduate students explained that they learned professional behaviour through their work with, and exposure to, senior professionals as well as through informal peer reflection. In one interview, for example, a graduating student spoke of learning to be a 'good' doctor as happening through experience observing and working with others:

The main thing is watching other people – clinical placements and being with other doctors. Picking out things you do want to do and things you don't want to do. Sometimes you think about it consciously and sometimes you are just absorbing it really and I think that is better than anything they can actually teach you in a lecture.

(Graduating Student)

Furthermore, and as the following extract illustrates, there was a sense that some of the undergraduate students also perceived that experience would be essential to their development as a good doctor:

I think life experience, if anything, is what will put me in good stead of being a good, when I say doctor I mean a good personable person. I think the course will help with the medical knowledge obviously but no, in terms of being a good doctor, in terms of the art of being a doctor, I think that's just life experience.

(Undergraduate Student)

Virtues of the 'ideal' doctor

In the survey respondents were again presented with the character strengths and, this time, were asked to rate the top six strengths of the 'ideal' doctor. The key finding in this regard was that the level of agreement between medical professionals at the three career stages about the top strengths required by the 'ideal' doctor was even greater than about the personal strengths reported above. Respondents in all three of the career stages – undergraduate students, graduate students and experienced doctors – placed the same character strengths in their top six[2]:

- fairness;
- honesty;
- judgement;
- kindness;
- leadership; and
- teamwork.

Four of these strengths – fairness, honesty, kindness and teamwork – were also in the five strengths selected most commonly by respondents across all three career stages as best reflecting their own personal character. Two – judgement and leadership – were not.

Table 3.2 shows the distribution of choices for each character strength. Similarly to the personal character strengths identified by

Table 3.2 Character strengths of the 'ideal' doctor

Figures in %	*Undergraduate students*	*Graduate students*	*Experienced doctors*
Appreciation of beauty	0	0	0
Bravery	1	1	1
Creativity	1	0	0
Curiosity	5	3	4
Fairness	7	7	9
Forgiveness	0	0	0
Gratitude	0	0	0
Honesty	12	15	14
Hope	1	1	1
Humour	1	1	3
Judgement	10	9	10
Kindness	10	11	10
Leadership	9	10	7
Love	1	1	0
Love of learning	6	6	7
Modesty	2	1	1
Perseverance	7	7	4
Perspective	4	5	4
Prudence	2	1	1
Self-regulation	3	3	6
Social intelligence	5	5	4
Spirituality	0	0	1
Teamwork	14	14	11
Zest	0	0	0
	100%	100%	100%

Table 3.3 The 'ideal' professional: three professions' views compared here

	Medicine	Law	Teaching
Number of common strengths identified (n)	6	5	5
Percentage of starting students identifying those common strengths as 'ideal' (%)	62	43	54
Percentage of graduating students identifying those common strengths as 'ideal' (%)	66	40	53
Percentage of experienced professionals identifying those common strengths as 'ideal' (%)	61	44	50

respondents, analysis of the data evidenced some differences based on respondents' gender. Most notably, female respondents were more likely to report judgement, kindness and leadership as strengths needed by the 'ideal' doctor than male respondents.

The degree of agreement amongst respondents about these qualities is striking, and is higher than the level of difference found in previous studies conducted by the Jubilee Centre on the legal (Arthur et al., 2014) and teaching (Arthur et al., 2015) professions. As set out in Table 3.3, across the three career stages, the same *six* common character strengths were selected as characterising the ideal doctor. While legal and teaching professionals at the three different career stages also demonstrated a high level of agreement on the common character strengths, such agreement in each study coalesced around five rather than six strengths. In addition, these six common character strengths in the medical practice study represented the choices of 62 per cent of undergraduate students, 66 per cent of graduates and 61 per cent of experienced professionals. These figures compare to a range of 40 to 44 per cent for students and practitioners of law and 50 to 54 per cent for student teachers and teachers. On the results of this analysis, it would seem that doctors at different stages of their career evidence a higher level of agreement on the character strengths important in the ideal doctor than do members of the legal and teaching professions.

To restate, analysis of the data found that respondents across the three career stages were consistent regarding the perceived character strengths of the 'ideal' doctor. This suggests a notable level of coherence regarding those qualities the good doctor should possess and exhibit. This is a doctor that is fair, honest, kind, shows leadership, works well as a team member and has good judgement. When the character strengths of the 'ideal' doctor were compared to the personal character strengths reported by respondents there was again a notable level of consistency. Overall the respondents in the study viewed themselves as possessing several of the character strengths similar to the ideal strengths they posited as required by doctors – fairness, honesty, kindness and teamwork. Developing this analysis further, the differences between the personal reported strengths respondents and those associated with the 'ideal' doctor are also notable with regard to the strengths of leadership and judgement. In the survey, respondents were more likely to report that leadership and judgement were strengths that should be possessed by the 'ideal' doctor than they were to report those as strengths they possess themselves (p < 0.05).

As might be expected, the interview data offered more nuanced accounts of how the respondents understood character in relation to their professional identify and practice. One of the themes emerging from the interview data, focused upon in the project report, was the view (also a key element of wider literature on virtue development) that the formation of professional character was not a finished or settled matter, but was in constant development. Experienced doctors, for example, pointed to the idea that doctors could not conceive of themselves as the 'finished product' but should rather 'strive to embody good character strengths' (Arthur et al., 2015: 17):

> *No, no one has the ideal set of characteristics to be the best doctor.*
> (Experienced Doctor)

> *I think that is the thing, being a doctor you are never a finished product.*
> (Experienced Doctor)

Clearly, such reflections point to the need for professionals to take a reflexive view of their work, including the moral elements of it, and of the importance of doctors having the time, spaces and structures that provide opportunities to be reflexive. This need was raised within a number of the interviews, with respondents often talking about the informal networks of support that help them to be reflexive, as the next extract demonstrates:

> *And then some of my friends who are GPs … You know, I talk a lot to them about – as doctors do – about interesting cases and ethical dilemmas and dilemmas with partners and employed staff at their practices, and I think I learn a lot from them and from their experiences, too.*
> (Experienced Doctor)

We return to such supportive mechanisms later in this chapter.

Two other themes that emerged in the interviews focused on influences on a doctor's character, namely those aspects of respondents' character that were viewed as more natural and, in addition, how experience shapes character. In the following extract, one respondent reflects on their own character in relation to their professional practice:

> *I think a huge part of [good character] is innate. Some people are ... I don't know, but certainly some of it is innate. You know, and I remember, you know, right as house officer, sort of within the first few weeks, you know, sitting up with the patient when I could have gone back to bed. Just sort of sitting and talking to her (...). But I think you get better at, certainly, things like – I'm in geriatric medicine now, so we do a lot of breaking bad news and sort of dealing with patients with dementia that sort of – dealing with families of people that are going to die .... So that, certainly, is an evolving skill.*
>
> (Experienced Doctor)

In explaining the core influences on their character as doctors, respondents at the different career stages spoke in varied ways about the importance of colleagues and role models in this regard.

Of further, and final, note here is the fact that in a meta-analysis of responses across a range of professions studied by the Jubilee Centre (Arthur et al., 2019), seven virtues were ranked highest in both the personal and professional domain:

- honesty;
- fairness;
- kindness;
- teamwork;
- perseverance;
- judgement; and
- leadership.

Of particular importance is that the five most commonly cited personal virtues (fairness, honesty, kindness, perseverance and team-work) and the six most commonly cited virtues associated with the 'ideal' doctor (fairness, honesty, kindness, teamwork, leadership and judgement) reported in the *Virtuous Medical Practice* study are all within this cross-professions list. That they are suggests that these virtues are common to all professions, though that does not necessarily mean that they hold the exact same meaning in each.

Virtues of the medical profession: the importance of context

No account of professional virtues can be considered even near complete if it does not speak to the context in which professionals act and practice. As the report on which this book is based made clear, 'the exercise of professional judgement does not occur in isolation ... but in wider social, political, economic and cultural contexts' (Arthur, 2015: 24), which highlight the importance of personal and moral dimensions of medical expertise in actual clinical situations (Bruce, 2007). As considered in earlier chapters of this book, the extant literature abounds with discussion about the ways in which organisational and work environments impact both positively and negatively on the formation and expression of character. Here we draw upon two sources of data to explore context. First, the e-survey data collected during the project, in particular a section of comprising 15 items exploring practising doctors' perceptions of their workplaces. This specific data subject to factor analysis, revealing four specific factors which the project team named 'autonomy', 'involvement', 'support' and 'challenge'. Second, interview data which explored respondents' perceptions of the influence of workplaces on their character, including the influence of medical regulation. Owing to the focus on workplaces influence and experiences, the data reported here comes solely from the experienced doctors in the sample.

Autonomy

Of the 15 questions in the e-survey, the following two questions – *I am able to act in the best interests of my patients* and *I have the resources to do my work to a standard I believe is right* – were found to factor together. The project team titled this factor 'autonomy' (see Table 3.4).

Table 3.4 Experienced doctors' views of the degree of autonomy they are accorded here

Factor 1: Autonomy N = 276 Mean = 3.86	Never to Rarely	Rarely to Sometimes	Sometimes to Mostly	Mostly to Always
	1–2	2.1–3	3.1–4	4.1–5
%	1.1	10.1	68.5	20.3

I am able to act in the best interests of my patients
I have the resources to do my work to a standard I believe is right

Of the 276 doctors who responded, 68.5 per cent reported that they practise with autonomy 'sometimes to mostly' and a further 20.3 per cent reported that they practice with autonomy 'mostly to always'. In the context of assertions of a loss of autonomy (see, for example, Andah et al., 2021) these findings present – at least on the surface – a more positive picture. On the other hand, of course, there may well be a difference at play between the actual level of autonomy (note the questions, for example, were 'I *am* able to act in the best interests of my patients' and 'I *have* the resources to do my work to a standard I believe is right') and the relative normative perceptions involved. In and of themselves, for example, the responses do not tell us whether the doctors believed themselves to have *sufficient* levels of autonomy (although this could more easily be read into the 'mostly to always' responses) or whether these levels had changed over a given period.

To gain a richer and more nuanced sense of these initial findings regarding autonomy we need again to consider the data garnered through the interviews. In the interviews, some respondents did indeed suggest that the autonomy of doctors had changed. For example, one doctor remarked that:

> *It used to be that doctors were gods. Now they have to conform to more national guidelines and if they don't, they're more likely to be caught out than they would have been years ago.*
>
> (Experienced Doctor)

While statements such as the above suggest change, they again only imply that change has happened – leaving open whether the change from the 'doctor as god' has been positive, negative or a mixture of both. In some of the interviews respondents spoke of wider changes in levels of autonomy while stating that in the context of their own work autonomy remained possible, if more constrained, within their professional practice. The following respondent, for example, spoke about their autonomous judgement:

> *I do feel that we're not allowed to use our judgement as much as we were previously. I do feel that the guidelines and policies are leading the way much more now … we have a lot of prescribing guidance, as I'm sure you're aware – a lot of places do – and there are a couple of medications that are classed as specialist only prescribing. But actually I do, in certain cases, prescribe them when I feel it is appropriate and I feel confident to actually undertake that prescribing and take the responsibility for it.*
>
> (Experienced Doctor)

Another respondent explained how decreasing levels of autonomy had paved the way for greater teamwork and collegiality, which in turn supported better judgements:

> *Less autonomy, which often people say that that's a bad thing, but actually I think a team approach to complex problems is really helpful. One of the things that is difficult when you qualify, particularly if you become a consultant or a GP, or once you reach a GP principal position or a consultant, is that you're expected to know everything and do everything and nobody ever watches you or listens to you in your practice ever again and therefore it's very easy to lose track and if you're making mistakes, not to necessarily realise them.*
>
> (Experienced Doctor)

In presenting these findings regarding autonomy we should also restate that the data in this section came from those respondents who were experienced doctors, and that doctors at much earlier stages of their career may encounter and reflect on professional autonomy in a different way. For instance, it may be the case that newly qualified doctors rely more heavily on algorithms and protocols to embed critical knowledge and to ensure patient safety (see Conroy et al., 2021 for further work on this question). In other words, the development of autonomous judgement (including the confidence to employ autonomous judgement) forms a core part of the learning process of being a doctor. As confidence grows with experience, clinicians feel more empowered to identify anomalies to patterns and therefore exercise autonomy using their clinical acumen. Appropriate deviation from protocol is a defining characteristic of expertise and expert performance (Ericsson et al., 2006).

Involvement

Factor analysis of the survey data found that another three questions in the e-survey factored together: *I am emotionally involved in my work*; *I have the feeling of doing useful work;* and *I am motivated to work to the best of my ability*. The original project team titled this factor 'involvement', with experienced doctors reporting a high degree of involvement in their work (see Table 3.5).

The experienced doctors tended to report high levels of involvement in their work. For example, 98.2 per cent responded that they are sometimes to mostly, or mostly to always, emotionally involved in their work,

Table 3.5 Experienced doctors' involvement in their work

Factor 2: Involvement N = 276 Mean = 4.10	Never to Rarely	Rarely to Sometimes	Sometimes to Mostly	Mostly to Always
	1–2	2.1–3	3.1–4	4.1–5
%	0	1.8	52.9	45.3

I am emotionally involved in my work
I have the feeling of doing useful work
I am motivated to work to the best of my ability

and only 1.8 per cent reported little or low emotional involvement in their work. Of course, while on the surface being 'involved' in one's work can be viewed as a positive, we must not rule out that for some high levels of emotional involvement in one's work as a doctor may not be wholly positive and runs the risk of emotional burnout.

The interviews provided the opportunity to dig deeper in order to understand influences on the levels of involvement that were at play – including those that inhibited the doctor's work. When experienced doctors spoke about the factors that were beneficial for their involvement in work, it was supportive colleagues that were emphasised most. As one of the experienced doctors interviewed explained:

> *The team that I'm in is fab. I like my partners all very much and I like the team that we've – you know, that we employ around us.*

Another experienced doctor also cited the importance of collegiality, identifying this alongside support from home as being of central importance in enabling them to work productively.

> *I think support from colleagues is a really, really important thing and also, therefore, support at home in terms of being – you've got to be happy at home to be able to do your job properly.*

Indeed, the home environment was a factor referred to frequently as helping doctors' involvement in their work. Often, the home environment was seen to play a crucial role in helping doctors to be able to be in the necessary cognitive and emotional condition needed for their work.

When interviewees turned to consider the factors that inhibited their level of involvement in their work two related issues stood out – workload and a lack of time to provide the level of appropriate care. Echoing other studies on the medical profession and on other professions, what came through in the interviews was a picture of the pressures of the working environments constraining doctors' work.

> *I guess time is always really the one you hear commonly mentioned, we have to battle against it, don't we? There are not enough hours in the day to do everything else to the true high standard that I would want to.*

(Experienced Doctor)

While not wishing to take anything away for the very real insights into the conditions in which the respondents were working, it is necessary to state that what also came through in some of the interviews was how the issues of workload and time were often tempered through and by a supportive environment. One of the respondents recounted the following experience, capturing how their home environment provided them with emotional care and sustenance:

> *I remember having sort of upwards of 50 patients that I had to see in one day. You're still seeing them in the afternoon, you can't do a good job, but actually, if you can come home to someone who's a human being and who actually loves you and doesn't sort of just say, yes, I know ... because I come home to someone who actually has a life outside of medicine, you know, who can sit there and understand, but actually can also tell me that there's a life outside of the stress and all the things that go on at work, but also listens to the facts of what I do.*

(Experienced Doctor)

Support

Returning to the e-survey, the importance of support was a further factor that arose out of the factor analysis, with the following give questions factoring together: *My colleagues help and support me*; *I am not treated fairly*; *I am able to apply my own ideas in my work*; *I am able to influence decisions that are important for my work;* and *I feel at home in my workplace.* Perhaps not surprisingly given the picture painted above in the interviews, levels of 'support' within the work environment met with mixed responses. As shown in Table 3.6, 65.9 per cent of doctors saw their working environment as sometimes to mostly supportive, with 24.6 per cent viewing it as mostly to always supportive, and 9.4 per cent saw their working environment as rarely providing support.

Table 3.6 Experienced doctors' view of the supportiveness of their work environment

Factor 3: Support N = 276 Mean = 3.76	Never to Rarely	Rarely to Sometimes	Sometimes to Mostly	Mostly to Always
	1–2	2.1–3	3.1–4	4.1–5
%	0.7	8.7	65.9	24.6

My colleagues help and support me
I am not treated fairly (scores reversed)
I am able to apply my own ideas in my work
I am able to influence decisions that are important for my work
I feel 'at home' in my workplace

Again, the interviews provided a more detailed account of how the experienced doctors' perceived their work environments. In this regard, issues such as targets and managerial pressures were identified as impacting negatively. One doctor, a GP, explicitly blamed service reconfigurations and funding cuts:

> *Support from your partners, very high educational standard in the practice that I work, in general a very good relationship with the patients, I think it's been hindered by NHS reconfigurations and current disinvestment in primary care.*

In one interview, an exchange developed within which the senior doctor told how they had relinquished a senior clinical management position because of the managerial pressures operating upon them:

EXPERIENCED DOCTOR: *I learnt whilst I was [deleted, job role], you've got to do what is right, whatever other people around you say and, if the people around you don't support you in doing what's right, you just stop doing it. You know, I mean, in the end, I stopped being the [job role] because the whole thing became incompatible with my value set.*

INTERVIEWER: *Really? I mean, could you say something briefly about that?*

EXPERIENCED DOCTOR: *Well, this is a few years ago now, but it was largely about managing fellow clinicians and I was told I was too nice, basically. I had to be more dictatorial.*

INTERVIEWER: *And if you had been, what end would that have achieved?*

EXPERIENCED DOCTOR: *Well, it would have perhaps, in the short term, got the outcome, the numbers would have stacked up and the target would have been hit, but ... [continues] ... if my relationship with my colleagues was so damaged as a result and I was therefore sort of excluded from, and I had behaved in a way that was persistently incompatible with my natural style, that was just too high a price really.*

Challenge

So far in this chapter we have, amongst other findings, reported how the respondents in the *Virtuous Medical Practice* study were actively balancing and managing their own conception of good medical practice with the supports and constraints experienced within and beyond the work environment. Five questions in the e-survey that factored together spoke to this balance and, more specifically to the ways that that work environment can force professionals, including doctors, to act against their moral character. Labelled 'challenge' by the original project team, the five questions in this area that factored together were: *My work involves tasks that are in conflict with my personal values; My work requires that I hide my feelings; I experience stress; At work it is difficult to do the right thing*; and *I do not have time to do my work to a standard I believe is right*. The analysis found that only 7.6 per cent of doctors rarely experience such challenge. While the majority of respondents, 70.3 per cent, experience such challenge only rarely to sometimes, a not insubstantial number (21.1 per cent) reported that they experience challenge to their personal moral character sometimes to mostly and 1.1 per cent mostly to always (see Table 3.7).

Table 3.7 Experienced doctors' perceptions of challenge to living out their character

Factor 4: Challenge N = 276 Mean = 2.75	Never to Rarely	Rarely to Sometimes	Sometimes to Mostly	Mostly to Always
	1–2	2.1–3	3.1–4	4.1–5
%	7.6	70.3	21.0	1.1

My work involves tasks that are in conflict with my personal values
My work requires that I hide my feelings
I experience stress
At work it is difficult to do the right thing
I do not have time to do my work to a standard I believe is right

Echoing some of the concerns already reported above, amongst the challenges the experienced doctors faced was how to respond appropriately to pressures of time, targets and budgets. The following experienced doctor explained that:

> *There have been times in the past where the way that things have been structured and the way funding has been, I felt that I've not been able to give patients the service I want. There was a time in [deleted] where, basically, orthopaedics didn't exist, there was such a long waiting list. Urgent cases were a year and I felt very frustrated that if I felt somebody needed an orthopaedic referral for something, that I was being blocked from that.*

The experienced doctor continued:

> *[When] you realise you're making decisions based on cost because you think: surely we're just going to do exactly what's the best thing for the patient. And then the reality of actually –, no, you need to actually look at what the costs are and that can be quite frustrating, so I suppose it's costs of tests that you want to do or costs of treatment, that's something that can be quite frustrating.*

In a similar vein, another experienced doctor spoke specifically about how pressures on time and workload impacted negatively on their ability to show patients compassion:

> *Actually it is quite easy, I think, in the sort of NHS we have now, you know, you have huge numbers of patients, you have very little time and actually it's quite easy to lose your compassion. It's not just compassion for the patients, but compassion for yourself, compassion for your colleagues and just the stress is such that actually you're not doing the job that you should be doing and actually, there's an interesting question about whether you can, given the number of patients.*

Of particular interest and importance here is not only that the culture and environment of the NHS places constraints on this doctor's conduct with their patients, but also their ability to practise self-compassion and compassion for their colleagues. That this is so speaks to the various pressures impacting on medical professionals as they seek to constantly mediate their own conceptions of being a 'good' doctor, the conceptions of others (including the profession itself) and the realities of professional life.

While here, and following the original project report (Arthur et al., 2015) we have drawn on the responses of experienced doctors to present medical professionals' experience of their workplace environments, we would also like to highlight that interaction between character and environment also came through at various times in the interviews with undergraduate students and graduating students. One of the latter, for example, suggested that:

> *I think, on the ward, so there's so much pressure that there's not actually all that much time to talk to patients, you know, to get through your jobs, so I think so long as I'm efficient and organised.*

(Graduating Student)

To view the relationship between character and workplace environment as straightforward would be over-simplistic. At times in the interview data, a picture is painted of the environment heavily constraining the sort of doctor respondents wanted to be. Yet, at other times – such as the example above – what comes across is not a denial of character, but the importance of character, even if it is of a more performance-focused kind (i.e. being efficient and organised). At other times still, and as we hope to have evidenced elsewhere in this chapter, what also comes across in the interview data not only that doctors are still able to express their moral character, but also that the pressures of time, workload and so on make this need ever more necessary.

Regulation

A fifth theme associated with the workplace that was identified by the project team was medical regulation. As Field suggests, 'health care professionals may feel that they spend more time complying with rules that direct their work than actually doing the work itself' (Field, 2008: 607). Similarly, Schwartz and Sharpe (2010) contend that the over-regulation of medical practice can be counter-productive. Although the e-survey did not specifically ask respondents about the impact of regulation on their professional work, in the interviews respondents were asked to share their thoughts on the guidelines that exist for ethical medical practice in the UK (such as The UK General Medical Council's (GMC, 2019) publication *Good Medical Practice*). When the interview data were analysed, differences between respondents at different stages of their career were evident. Notably, first year students tended to regard *Good Medical Practice* as a document to adhere to strictly. One medical educator reported how their students frequently saw the document as directing doctor's work:

> *The first years sometimes come to me and say, 'The GMC says ...'*
> *it's 'these are the things that I know I have to do or not do', and it isn't*
> *internal at any way, shape or form at that point.*

In contrast, graduating students tended to speak of the document in more nuanced terms, viewing *Good Medical Practice* as providing partial guidance that needed to be moderated in some ways by context and judgement. For example, one graduating student explained that:

> *I was actually reading through it yesterday, it does, but I think what*
> *I like best is you have more, I don't know if there's access to sort of*
> *examples, where you put the guidelines into practice, 'cause some-*
> *times when you're reading something through, it's difficult to gauge*
> *exactly what they're trying to get and to sort of think in your head, oh,*
> *if this now happened, is this what they'd want me to do.*
>
> (Graduate Student)

Importantly, across the experienced doctors various approaches and relationships to the guidelines were reported. While some respondents explained that they had not read the document for some time, what really came through in these interviews was a sense that each professional had developed, and was developing, ongoing ways of working with key guidelines – and that these varied between respondents. There is not space here to give full expression to the responses. However, the following extracts give a sense of the general picture:

> *So, I've always seen* Good Medical Practice *as ... having it on the*
> *desk beside me if I'm ... you know, evolving a project or something*
> *like that.*
>
> (Experienced Doctor)

> *I think they must do [have an influence], even subconsciously, or*
> *because – I don't think there's anything there that's either alarming*
> *or surprising, in the GMC guidance, so ... But then, it's some-*
> *thing there to refer to if you're sort of reminding yourself what – I*
> *suppose, what the specifics are ... Does it influence my practice on*

a day-to-day level? I don't think I consciously think, on a day-to-day level, 'Oh, I'd better not do that because it's not in the GMC guidance.' I think that I think … It's a step before that, isn't it? It's about what I think is a reasonable person or a reasonable doctor going to do in this situation.

(Experienced Doctor)

The GMC is the Daily Mail of the medical profession, they are interested in the reputation of the medical profession and how it looks on the outside. They don't care, individually, of the individual doctor. You have to, in their eyes, a good doctor, you know, is an advertisement for the profession, he has to demonstrate and be seen to be a good role model for the profession, so yes, it's a reputation PR sort of organisation.

(Experienced Doctor)

I don't necessarily think about GMC guidelines every day but only because I think my practice runs pretty much within them, and if it was ever to – if I was ever to do anything that might even slightly come into conflict with any of it, then I would start thinking about it.

(Experienced Doctor)

Furthermore, the experienced doctors conveyed the view that while professional guidance *informs* medical practice, it does not and cannot *replace* professional knowledge and the virtue of moral judgement. It should be noted, of course, that the understanding and use of the guidance taken by the experienced doctors is recognised by the GMC and features within the guidance itself, which addressing doctors directly states that doctors are expected 'to use your professional judgement and expertise to apply the principles in this guidance to the various situations you face'.[3] This general view was also conveyed within the interviews with the medical educators, one of whom offered the following interpretation, which speaks to the importance of context, application and learning from experience:

I think the GMC's guidance is there as a kind of bottom line I think rather than, I mean, if you just went to medical school and spent 5 years just reading GMC guidelines, it's not going to teach you how to be a good doctor. I think it's there to tell you what the boundaries are rather than as being a guide as to how to practice. And as I say, the guidance on how to practice doesn't exist, because it's age old, it's watching previous generations of doctors, working alongside them and learning it by experience really.

(Medical Educator)

Another medical educator also highlighted the importance of experience and judgement (broadly akin to *professional phronesis*, though they did not use that specific term) in discerning the right course of action in a given situation:

When you're looking at the GMC's guidance, a lot of it, it's just detailed, but yet actually if you were a doctor and you had a particular scenario, very often that scenario is not covered, so it's not, even though it's quite long, it's not actually that precise … They also use Good Medical Practice, you know those interactive case studies … [continues] and then they say at the end, but don't take this as any statement that this is indicative of the law and you think, well, how flipping helpful is that, not at all.

(Medical Educator)

Before we finish, one further point is worth noting here. This is that in the interviews with the experienced doctors some identified greater regulation as having *positive* impacts. Speaking about regulatory practices involved in their work, one of the experienced doctors reflected:

I think, while there's been lots of negative change in the medical profession, this might actually be one that over the last few years has perhaps changed for the positive, because there is actually, much as we dislike it, but there is actually more kind of appraisal of what we do whereas, you know, 20 or 30 years ago GPs in particular could practice in pretty much isolation and hardly anyone used to check on what they were doing … unless there was something majorly going wrong, whereas now with appraisal and with other forms of assessments, say with the Care Quality Commission coming in, I guess we are more and more having to ask ourselves, you know, is the way we do things right, have we got the right protocols in place and also, you know, reflect more on our decision making so it's probably, I hesitate to say this, it probably is getting better.

To conclude this section, and as we have suggested previously, the argument that codes of professional ethics do not provide a sufficient basis for informing and guiding professional conduct is not the same as saying that such codes do not play a necessary part. Instead, codes of professional conduct provide part of the picture, but do so as one constituent alongside others that comprise the basis of the varied deliberations doctors undertake in seeking to be good professionals. In other words, professional wisdom develops over time in a professional context as practising clinicians interact with colleagues, patients, families, processes, guidelines and other salient factors within complex settings.

Conclusion

The data presented and analysed in this chapter provides an indication of how medical professionals at different stages of their career perceive their personal character strengths as doctors and the character strengths equated with the 'ideal' or 'good' doctor. The data paints a picture of doctors at different stages of their career prioritising certain core virtues as central to their own work and those of the doctors they aspire to be – fairness, honesty, kindness, teamwork, leadership, perseverance, and judgement. Mirroring existing literature in the field, we have also drawn on the responses of doctors across the career stages to consider what it takes to realise these virtues in practice, including the very real and pervasive constraints that can prevent doctors from fully fulfilling the moral dimensions of their work. In this regard, the data reported here portrays medical professionals as carefully traversing complex and challenging workplace environments within which they mediate their vision of the ideal medical professional, their personal characteristics, relevant regulations, time and workload pressures, and – crucially – the needs of their patients. What comes through are contexts within which doctors express and enact character, but in which their ability to do so is constrained by the varied pressures placed upon them. In navigating this terrain, professional wisdom is essential. In addition, and within such environments, doctors are often sustained in their work by supportive teams, colleagues and families. Indeed, while not wishing to diminish the very real burdens and constraints upon doctors at the various stages of their careers in any shape or form, we must not lose sight of the fact that, constrained as it may be, doctors are enacting the moral dimensions of their work on a daily basis, informed and guided by their professional wisdom. This reflection is not only relevant for current doctors, but for those entering the profession. We chose to end this chapter with the following account drawn from an interview with a Graduating Student in which they recounted the inspirational work of doctors observed as part of their studies:

Some of the things that stand out are some of the doctors when they are breaking bad news, how people do that. I've seen one GP who did that very well, an oncology consultant who did that really, really well. And I had a big discussion afterwards with him. He said how difficult it was, how he does it and after that he went to a meeting and discussed it with colleagues. That helped him deal with his emotions about it. His main character strengths were being able to show the patient that he really empathised with them but could still remain professional. It obviously affected him but he managed not to show that too much but he showed how much he felt for them and gave them the opportunity to ask questions and didn't overload them with information and things.

(Graduating Student)

Notes

1 With 24 items to choose from, the top six do not account for all choices and one item from a set of six can only amount to a maximum of 16.7 per cent of all choices. Thus, if 'honesty' represents 11 per cent of all choices by experienced doctors (see Table 3.1), it means 66 per cent of experienced doctors selected that item as one of their top six personal strengths.

2 It should be noted here that, in actuality, it may be the case that the specific ratings differ based on the medical practitioners' specialities. In the study there were not sufficiently large sub-cohorts of specialities to test this hypothesis for the sample.

3 www.gmc-uk.org/ethical-guidance/ethical-guidance-for-doctors/good-medical-practice.

4 Medical practitioners, ethical dilemmas and the perspectives of medical educators

Introduction

Drawing on data collected by the *Virtuous Medical Practice* project, analysis is presented of responses to a series of ethical dilemmas given to the medical students and experienced doctors. Across a number of Jubilee Centre projects, moral dilemmas have been used as a data collection tool (Arthur et al., 2014; 2015b; 2018; Kristjánsson et al., 2017). In the *Virtuous Medical Practice* study, participants responded to a set of professional dilemmas (six situational judgement tests (Patterson and Ashworth, 2011; Lievens and Patterson, 2011) designed by a panel of 15 experts in medical education who adapted well-known dilemmas from the literature and designed a wholly new set of answer responses specifically for the study). As explained in the introduction to this book, dilemmas were used as they (a) promise to offer a credible way to gain an insight into moral functioning and development, and (b) can ideally be designed so as to activate more than simply moral reasoning skills (Kristjánsson, 2015, chap. 3; see also Gardiner, 2003). These benefits noted, it is important to clarify that responses to dilemmas serve as an indication, rather than guarantee, of action or understanding of moral sensitivity in a real, particular situation. They do not, in and by themselves, *measure* virtue, nor do any such definitive measures exist elsewhere. Rather, when combined with data from interviews and self-reports dilemmas may contribute to an overall understanding of virtue in professional practice.

The intention in employing the six dilemmas was not to seek a certain, pre-determined 'correct' response from respondents, but was instead to ask respondents to explain their reasoning and the judgements arrived at with a particular focus on virtue-based reasoning. It was hoped that the situational judgement tests would give us an insight into: (a) which character strengths are important in dilemma situations in medicine; (b) how; and (c) how they interact with other factors, such as explicit

DOI: 10.4324/9781003137887-5

rules for medical practice and the consequences of certain decisions.[1] Each of the dilemmas focused on a particular challenge that raised professional demands. The use of dilemmas as a research instrument reflects the fact that 'professionals may face workplace dilemmas where they are required to make decisions that conflict with the desires of external agents' (Arthur et al., 2019; see also Moore, 2015). Such dilemmas take many forms, of course, no least in their seriousness and precise contours. Responding to dilemmas is, of course, a frequent requirement of professional life. As an experienced doctor stated in their interview 'ethical dilemmas turn up constantly':

> *I don't think there's a day goes by without some kind of, you know, ethical decision.*
>
> (Experienced Doctor)

As we have suggested earlier in this book, this regular engagement with various complex dilemmas – often where medical professionals are concerned dilemmas that are matters of life and death – requires professionals to possess and enact core intellectual virtues commensurate with professional wisdom, including judgement/prudence and perspective, in order to discern the morally good course of action in the given circumstances (Carr, 2018). We contend that considering dilemmas can offer important insights into how medical professionals engage with a problem, and that we can learn something about their deliberation processes.

The chapter comprises three main sections. In the first, we detail and analyse the findings in relation to three of the six dilemmas respondents were asked to consider. Based on the associations made by the expert panel, each of these three dilemmas incorporated a conflict between different virtues. In the analysis we point to the differences across and between the three career stages in terms of the chosen course of action, as well as to the reasons selected (from a pre-given list) for these choices. In the second section, we look at the data across the dilemmas to report how reasons prioritised give a picture of the virtues at play (on the basis of associations between reasons and specific virtues made by the expert panel). In addition, the responses to the dilemmas provide additional data regarding the role of professional codes of conduct in doctors' reasoning about the dilemmas, once again demonstrating how rules and virtues often combine in ethical decision-making. In the third section, we seek to add further depth to the findings and analysis presented in this chapter (and indeed the previous chapter) by exploring key themes raised in the interviews with medical educators.

Moral dilemmas and character strengths

Here, we focus in some detail on the responses to *three* of the six dilemmas engaged with by respondents that individually, and taken together, illustrate how for the respondents in the study virtues operate both in concord and in conflict.[2] In addition, the responses to the three dilemmas were chosen because they provide an insight into how the virtues of the 'ideal' doctor examined in the previous chapter work together in practice, and how reasons concerned with virtues and, in some notable cases, rules for conduct, influence medical students' and doctors' moral decision-making in relation to the dilemmas.

Dilemma: a conflict between kindness and leadership

The first dilemma we analyse here (Dilemma 5 in the study) asked respondents to consider what they would do in the following situation:

> *You are a junior doctor on call at a local hospital. A colleague arrives at the hospital to take over from you, smelling of alcohol. This is not the first time this colleague has arrived at work smelling of alcohol.*

Respondents were given two possible responses from which to choose. Option 1 was that they would speak to their colleague privately. Option 2 was that they would speak to the supervising consultant. Based on their choice of either option 1 or 2, respondents were then provided with six reasons that could justify their choice of option, and were asked to rank the answers that best matched their reasons. For those respondents who reported that they would speak to the colleague privately (option 1), the following six reasons were offered:

Reason 1: You want to maintain a friendly professional relationship with your colleague.

Reason 2: You are concerned about your colleague and want to help him/her.

Reason 3: You want to give him/her a chance to explain and improve.

Reason 4: You want to try and resolve the issue without getting formally involved.

Reason 5: You are following *General Medical Council* guidance.

Reason 6: You are trying to solve the problem without damaging the career of your colleague.

For those respondents who reported that they would speak to the supervising consultant (option 2), the following six reasons were offered:

Reason 1: You want to avoid potentially harmful consequences for patient safety.

Reason 2: There may be risks for you personally if you do not report him/her.

Reason 3: It is not your responsibility to deal directly with your colleague.

Reason 4: NHS policy encourages whistleblowing – you would be following guidance.

Reason 5: No harm will be done to your professional relationship with your colleague, as you will report him/her confidentially.

Reason 6: You will protect your colleague's reputation.

63 per cent of respondents reported that they would choose to speak to their colleague privately (option 1), with 37 per cent reporting that they would speak to the supervising consultant (option 2). When the data were analysed with respect to respondents at different stages of their careers, some notable differences between the three cohorts emerged regarding how likely they would be to speak to a supervising consultant about the colleague. Whereas 48 per cent of experienced practitioners and 42 per cent of first-year undergraduate students selected this option, only 15 per cent of graduating students responded that they would speak to the supervising consultant. The fact that 85 per cent of graduating students would deal with the matter privately (compared with 58 per cent of first-year students and 52 per cent of experienced doctors) seems striking. Given that the method employed in the study did not permit space for detailed dialogue with the graduating students about why they would choose this option, we have to look instead to other considerations to seek to make sense of this finding. In this regard, the ranked reasons given for each of the options were informative.

For those respondents who chose option 1, reason 2 – *You are concerned about your colleague and want to help him/her* – was the both the most frequent reason selected and the most frequent *first* reason chosen (remembering that each respondent ranked their three chosen options). The expert panel who designed the dilemmas were of the opinion that this reason, if chosen, would point to the virtue of kindness amongst respondents. The second most selected reason was reason 3 – *You want to give him/her a chance to explain and improve*, which the expert panel

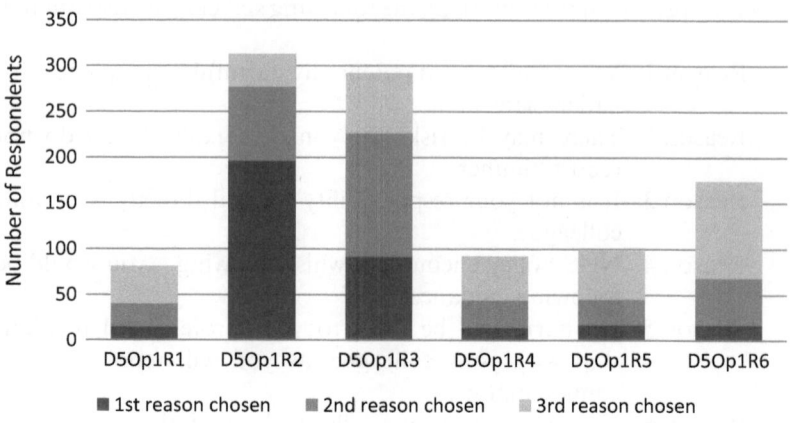

Chart 4.1 Dilemma 5 option 1 – all respondents.

categorised as indicating the virtue of fairness or perspective. The third most selected reason was reason 6 – *You are trying to solve the problem without damaging the career of your colleague.* As with reason 2, the expert panel took to this reason as drawing upon the virtue of kindness. Those three reasons least selected were reasons 1, 4 and 5 (in that order). The expert panel considered that these, respectively, were suggestive of wanting to work as a team with the colleague (reason 1), a concern with mere consequences (reason 4) and a concern to follow General Medical Council guidance (reason 5). Chart 4.1 shows the results for all three career groups in choosing option 1 for dilemma 5.

Returning more specifically to the difference in responses by the graduating students, who were far more likely to report that they would speak to the colleague than first-year students and experienced doctors, the project team learnt that many of the graduating students had recently been taught, as part of their studies, to try and deal with matters such as the one in the dilemma privately in the first instance. This may, of course, have influenced the differential found. Though we cannot be certain of their motives, we cannot rule out that the choices may also reflect that as new entrants to the profession they were acutely aware that newly qualified doctors often work long hours and in relative isolation. It could be the case that, in such conditions, these respondents were signifying that they would be more compassionate to the colleague on this basis – seeking to appeal directly to them in the first instance. Whatever was the actual reason, the graduating students as a group did not offer a mere rule or convention as the reason why they would choose to speak to their colleague privately in the first instance.

Turning now to the reasons selected by those respondents who chose option 2 – to speak to the supervising consultant – there was a high level of agreement as to *why* they would do so. Reason 1 – *You want to avoid potentially harmful consequences for patient safety* was both the most frequently given reason and the reason most frequently ranked as the most important reason behind the option. Notably, all but one respondent (99.5 per cent of respondents) included this reason in their three choices of reasons and almost all ranked it first. The expert panel connected this reason to the virtues of leadership and judgement. The next most frequently chosen reasons by those respondents opting to speak to the supervising consultant were reason 4 – *NHS policy encourages whistleblowing – you would be following guidance* and reason 6 – *You will protect your colleague's reputation*. The expert panel were of the view that these reasons point to concerns with following the rules (reason 4) and with kindness, teamwork or forgiveness (reason 6). From these responses, it seems clear that when there are clear rules or policies that guide how professionals should behave, direct appeal to such rules is offered by a large number of respondents as the reason for their choice. Given this, two reflections seem important. First, and more directly, rules and codes of conduct can and do play an important role in shaping doctors' thinking about morally challenging situations including in situations where professional virtues – such as judgement and kindness – are at play. Indeed, for the following respondent the sorts of considerations central to a virtue-based approach to professionalism and professional practice were captured *within* the protocols involved:

> *I have seen sorts of conflicts but I think there's so many sort of protocol and guidelines, but so long as you know those for a particular situation, then I think there's little room for the personal values. I think it can make it more difficult to manage a patient, but I think for most things there are clear guidelines with how you should behave and why you would have to justify if you weren't going to follow that protocol ... I think looking at the patient and making them more comfortable is always the most important thing and whatever is in the best interest of the patient is always the most important thing. I think that's usually at the centre of most of the guidelines anyway.*
>
> (Experienced Doctor)

Second, and more tentatively, there is a possibility that the type of dilemma (i.e. what is precisely at stake) may well lead to different

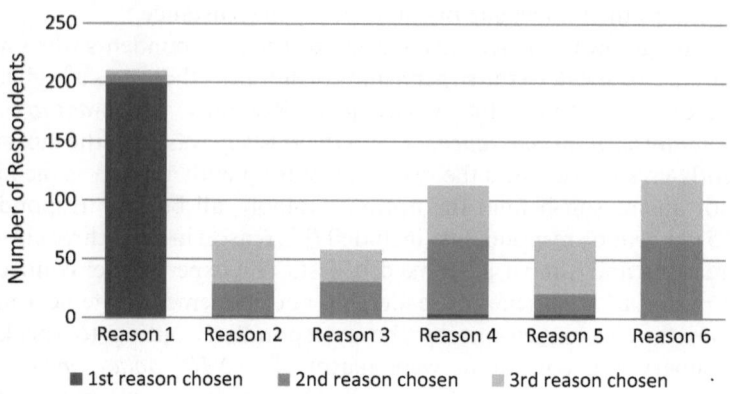

Chart 4.2 Dilemma 5 option 2 – all respondents.

emphasis being placed on particular reasons. For example, in their interview, one of the graduating students reflected in relation to the importance of their personal beliefs:

> *I think it depends how much of a conflict it is. If it's just something smaller then I'd compromise on my personal beliefs straight away and do what's right for the profession. But if it's something I strongly dis-agreed with I think I'd have to reflect on it before I took it any further and maybe talk to some seniors about it or something.*
>
> (Graduating Student)

More research is needed to uncover whether this tentative suggestion is actually the case more generally (i.e. whether the particular dynamics and the perceived 'stakes' of the dilemma in question impacts on the sorts of reasons selected). Chart 4.2 shows the results for all three career groups in choosing option 2 for dilemma 5.

Dilemma: a conflict between using one's judgement, prudence and rules

In the second dilemma (Dilemma 4 in the study) we analyse here, respondents were asked how they would respond to the following situation:

> *You have just taken over a single-handed general practice in a small, isolated community. You have always wanted a rural practice, and hope someday to marry and raise children there. Pat Cuthbert is an attractive, intelligent, level-headed patient whose family has lived in*

the community for generations. Pat is also a member of the hiking club you have joined. You have been treating Pat for some time for a skin condition, which appears to be clearing up. Although visits will continue to be necessary for monitoring, the patient is substantially improved. At the end of a visit, Pat smiles warmly and invites you to dinner, clearly showing an interest in being more than your patient.

Respondents were given two options. Option 1 – accept the invitation or Option 2 – do not accept the invitation.

As with the dilemma above, respondents were given six reasons for each of the options and were asked to rank the three reasons that best matched their decision. For Option 1 – accept the invitation – the following six reasons were provided:

Reason 1: You find Pat attractive.
Reason 2: You are already seeing Pat socially.
Reason 3: You would like to start a serious relationship.
Reason 4: Everyone you meet will be your patient; this dilemma will keep arising in a setting like this.
Reason 5: There won't be any harm in it.
Reason 6: You don't want to appear rude by refusing.

For Option 2 – do not accept the invitation – the following six reasons were provided:

Reason 1: This is what is suggested by the 'Good Medical Practice' guidelines.
Reason 2: You want to preserve the professional doctor–patient relationship.
Reason 3: Your career may be damaged if this gets out.
Reason 4: Gossip and even scandal may ensue.
Reason 5: You may end up in an awkward situation if the relationship does not work.
Reason 6: Conflicts may arise with other patients.

When the data were analysed the results evidenced that a large majority of the respondents (84 per cent) reported that they *would not* accept the invitation, although experienced professionals were slightly more inclined to accept the invitation compared to starting undergraduates and completing graduates. For example, whereas 20 per cent of experienced professionals reported that they *would* accept such an invitation, only 13 per cent of students selected the same option

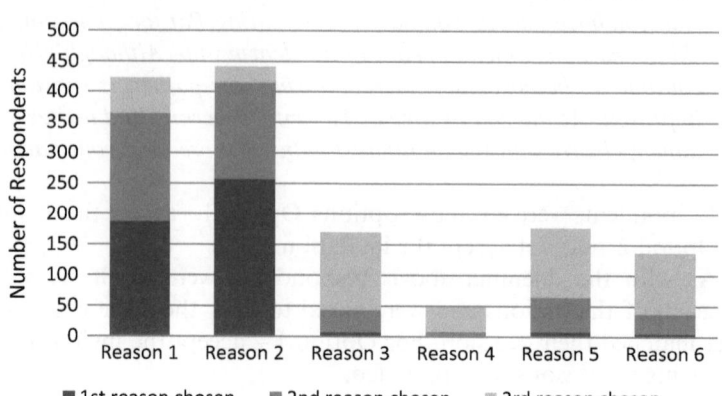

Chart 4.3 Dilemma 4 option 2 – all respondents.

($p < 0.05$). Male respondents were significantly more likely to choose option one (that is, to take up the invitation) than female respondents ($p < 0.05$).

The reason that most respondents gave as to why they would *not* become personally involved with a patient was reason 2 – *You want to preserve the professional doctor-patient relationship.* According to the expert panel, reason 2 points to the importance of prudence for the practitioner. Next most frequently selected was reason 1, *This is what is suggested by the 'Good Medical Practice' guidelines.* There was no clear third reason. Chart 4.3 shows the results for all three career groups in choosing option 2 for dilemma 4. In thinking through the selection of these two reasons, and as highlighted by the original project team (Arthur et al., 2015), it is apparent that the two most selected reasons involve what the expert panel considered to be a virtue-based reason (the good of the doctor–patient relationship) and a rule-based reason (following the GMC guidelines). Moreover, for these respondents, the two reasons were very closely matched as to their importance.

Amongst the 16 per cent of respondents ($n = 88$) who indicated they would accept the invitation, reason 4 – *Everyone you meet will be your patient; this dilemma will keep arising in a setting like this* was the most selected choice, and was also the first choice for most of the respondents. The second most frequently chosen reason was reason 2 – *You are already seeing Pat socially*, while reason 3 – *You would like to start a serious relationship* – was the third most selected reason (and was

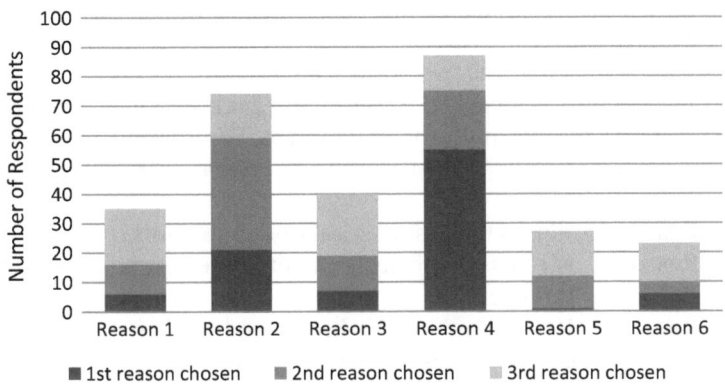

Chart 4.4 Dilemma 4 option 1 – all respondents.

mostly selected as the third of the three ranked reasons). When the associations drawn for each reason as adjudicated by the expert panel are considered, these reasons point to character strengths such as: perspective or judgement (reason 4), kindness (reason 2) and hope (reason 3). The reasons least often chosen were those to do with consequences or social expectations. Reason 5, *There won't be any harm in it*, and reason 6, *You don't want to appear rude by refusing* were, respectively, the second least and the least selected reasons. Chart 4.3 shows the results for all three career groups in choosing option 1 for dilemma 4.

Dilemma: a conflict between prudence, rules and respect

In the third dilemma (Dilemma 1 in the study) we analyse here, the respondents were presented with the following dilemma:

> *You are a GP, and are called out on a home visit to an 87 year old patient – Mr G. – who you have not met before. From his patient history, you see that he has an existing heart condition. You find him experiencing severe chest pains and shortness of breath, as well as low blood pressure. During your assessment, he appears to be deteriorating. You judge that he is having a heart attack, and that there is a strong chance he may die soon. You believe the best option would be to admit him to hospital immediately. However, despite extensive explanations from you, Mr G. is adamant he does not want to go to the hospital but wants to stay in his own home.*

Respondents were given two options from which to select: Option 1 – admit Mr G. to hospital and Option 2 – Don't admit Mr G. to hospital, and arrange end-of-life care at home.

Again, for each of the two options a set of six reasons were provided and respondents were asked to select and rank the three answers that best matched the reasons for their decisions. For option 1 – *you chose to admit Mr G. to hospital* – the following six reasons were given:

Reason 1:   This is the best medical option for Mr G.
Reason 2:   Mr G. is distressed and not in the best position to make this decision.
Reason 3:   If you don't admit Mr G. and he dies, you might face consequences in the Coroner's Court.
Reason 4:   Your diagnosis may not be correct and you don't want to take the chance with Mr G.'s life.
Reason 5:   If Mr G. dies you will feel guilty for not having done all you could to save him.
Reason 6:   This is what GPs are expected to do.

For option 2 – *you chose not to admit Mr G. to hospital* – the following reasons were given:

Reason 1:   You should respect Mr G. by accepting his wishes.
Reason 2:   Mr G. is quite likely to die anyway, so he may as well be allowed to stay at home.
Reason 3:   Trying to treat Mr G. against his own wishes isn't the best use of the hospital's resources.
Reason 4:   You are confident you will be able to give effective end-of-life care for Mr G. at home.
Reason 5:   This is the kindest option for Mr G.
Reason 6:   Professional guidance states that if the patient is capable you should comply with their wishes

82 per cent of the respondents selected option 2 – *Don't admit Mr G. to hospital*. While this option was selected by over 60 per cent of respondents in each of the three career stages, there was a notable difference between the career stages, with the proclivity to select this option rising with experience. 90 per cent of experienced doctors reported that they would *not* admit Mr G. to hospital, the option selected by 83 per cent of graduating students. Of the first year undergraduate students, however, 63 per cent reported that they would not admit Mr G. Conversely, only 18 per cent of respondents said that they would

admit Mr G. to hospital. This option was chosen by 37 per cent of the undergraduates, 17 per cent of the graduates and 10 per cent of the experienced professionals in the sample.

Turning to the reasons selected for the two options, the most frequently selected reasons by the respondents who *would* admit Mr G. were reasons 1 – *This is the best medical option for Mr G.* and reason 2 – *Mr G. is distressed and not in the best position to make this decision.* Taken together, reasons 1 and 2 represented 68 per cent of all choices across all career stages. Reason 1 was categorised by the expert panel as pointing to the virtues of prudence, judgement, kindness or even leadership on the part of respondents, while the expert panel aligned reason 2 with the virtue of judgement. The reasons that were least often chosen were reason 6 – *This is what GPs are expected to do* – and reason 3 – *If you don't admit Mr G. and he dies, you might face consequences in the Coroner's Court.* The expert panel regarded reason 6 as reflecting a rules-based approach (or at least a conventional approach) and reason 3 as reflecting a consequences-based approach. Chart 4.5 shows the results for all three career groups in choosing option 1 for dilemma 1.

Moving to the majority of the participants (82 per cent) who reported that they would *not* admit Mr G. to hospital, the most frequently cited reasons were reason 1 – *You should respect Mr G. by accepting his wishes* and reason 6 – *Professional guidance states that if the patient is capable you should comply with their wishes.* The expert panel judged reason 1 as indicating the virtues of kindness and bravery, and reason 6 as signifying following a given rule for action. The least frequently chosen reasons were reason 3 – *Trying to treat Mr G. against his own wishes isn't the best use of the hospital's resources* and reason 2 – *Mr G. is*

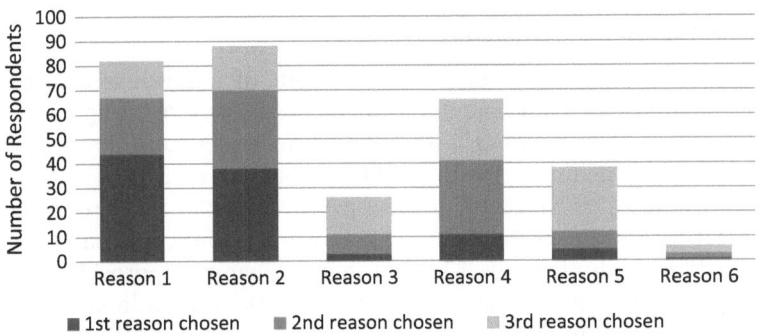

Chart 4.5 Dilemma 1 option 1 – all respondents.

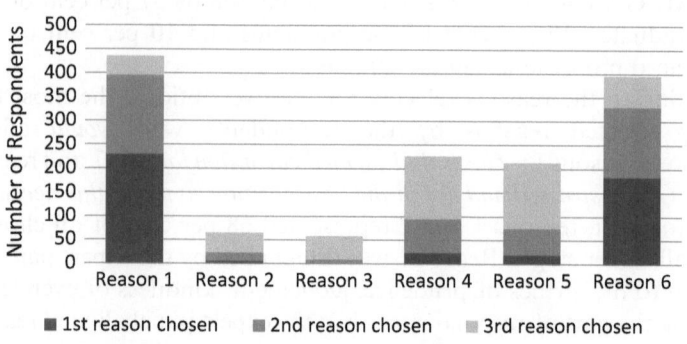

Chart 4.6 Dilemma 1 option 2 – all Respondents.

quite likely to die anyway, so he may as well be allowed to stay at home.
Chart 4.6 shows the results for all three career groups in choosing
Option 2 for dilemma 1.

For the respondents who would not admit Mr G. to hospital, the
reasons concerned with respecting Mr G.'s wishes and the desire to
follow explicit guidance were closely matched in terms of the importance accorded to them. Once again, with this dilemma the reasons given
for the most popular option seemed to prioritise a virtue-focused consideration (in this case the kindness or bravery involved in taken the
option of not admitting Mr G. to hospital (with the risk in terms of
his survival chances) and a rule-based consideration. There remains the
suggestion here that for the respondents taking this option, character
and professional guidance operate in concert in informing the decision
selected.

Looking across the dilemmas

In this section we set out some key points of analysis offered by the
original project team, and add our own analysis in looking across the
dilemmas. The dilemmas were designed to understand how considerations of virtue interact with thinking about rules and consequences in
the responses provided by medical professionals at the three different
career stages. From the discussion above, it should be clear that it is
possible to adopt the well-known moral dilemma approach to focus,
not only on moral reasoning, but to explore additional considerations concerning virtue, such as motivational and emotional factors.

While the dilemmas cannot capture all of the contextual and agent-based nuances of real life, they were designed by the expert panel to capture pertinent quandaries and conflicts. The most fruitful way to think of moral dilemmas, then, from a virtue-perspective is to conceive of such dilemmas as situations in which different virtues – and, sometimes, virtues and rules – come into conflict. According to traditional virtue ethics, that is exactly when *phronesis*, or practical wisdom, is most needed. Here, two key considerations stand out. First, that being motivated by *a* virtue does not in itself guarantee moral rightness if it is not *the* virtue appropriate for the specific context. Second, that situations exist in which two virtues conflict, meaning that in these situations the professional will need to prioritise one or more virtues, without necessarily discounting others fully. This is the role of *phronesis*, to adjudicate and integrate virtue, emotion and cognition with an orientation towards morally guided action.

In addition, the data gathered in relation to the dilemmas provides some additional insights into *which* virtues played a role in shaping the respondents' choices – an important part of the exploratory aims with the research. The first point to note here, which was reported by the original project team (Arthur et al., 2015) was that in evaluating the moral dilemmas, the expert panel mapped the reasons for action provided to specific virtues. That is, the expert panel indicated which of the 24 virtue words from the Peterson and Seligman classification (also used in sections 1 and 3 of the survey) could be associated with the specific reasons for choosing the given options in each of the 6 dilemmas. In specifying these virtues, the expert panel drew heavily on only a small number of virtues out of the list of 24. The frequency of the 'mapped' virtues to reasons is shown in Table 4.1.

The frequencies in this table indicate that, in *their* thinking about the moral dilemmas, the expert panel identified the virtues of judgement, kindness, fairness, prudence, leadership and perspective as being highly relevant matters that could potentially shape a doctor's thinking about the range of moral dilemmas used in the study. This offers additional weight to the findings reported in Chapter 3 regarding the importance of the virtues of judgement, kindness, fairness and leadership for medical professionals.

In addition, the virtues associated by the expert panel with the reasons most frequently selected by respondents are also of note. Table 4.2 illustrates the number of times reasons mapped to particular character strengths were selected by respondents (1) in their top three choices and (2) as their first choice.

Table 4.1 Character strengths used by the expert panel in the dilemmas here

Character Strength	Number of times the expert panel mapped this strength against a particular reason for action
Judgement	21
Kindness	13
Fairness	10
Prudence	10
Leadership	8
Perspective	8
Bravery	6
Teamwork	4
Social intelligence	3
Hope	3
Self-regulation	2
Curiosity	2
Humility	1
Perseverance	1
Appreciation of beauty	1
Love	1
Forgiveness	1

The remaining virtues from the list of 24 were not used by the expert panel at all.

Table 4.2 Character strengths selected by respondents in the dilemmas

Character Strength	Number of times an item mapped to this strength was selected by respondents in the top 3 choices	Number of times an item mapped to this strength was selected by respondents as the first choice
Judgement	13	6
Kindness	11	6
Fairness	7	3
Leadership	6	3
Prudence	4	3
Bravery	4	1
Perspective	4	1
Social intelligence	2	1

This data indicates, once more in accordance with the findings presented in Chapter 3, that respondents were inclined to select the reasons that the expert panel associated with the virtues of judgement, kindness, fairness and leadership. Three different sources of information, then, point to the importance of the virtues of judgement, kindness, fairness and leadership in the ethical practice of medicine:

- respondents' reported views of the character of the 'ideal' doctor;
- a group of medical educators' judgement of which virtues are in play in moral dilemma situations in medicine; and
- respondents' choices amongst the reasons for acting one way or another in the situational judgement tests on the e-survey.

Overall, the responses to the dilemmas point to a widespread reliance not only on virtue-based considerations, but considerations involving a small group of commonly favoured virtues. Rule-based considerations are also common, often complementing rather than contradicting virtue-based reasons. Notably, too, considerations of consequences or utility were rarely given preference.

Medical educators and medical education

To this point in the book, we have largely considered the views of the medical students and experienced doctors who participated in the *Virtuous Medical Practice* study. On occasion we have supplemented these views with extracts from the interviews with the sample of medical educators (n = 10) who were also interviewed. Recalling from the introduction to this book that an important element of the study was to illicit the views of medical educators, and to consider their practice at the time, in this final section we report on some key themes of the interviews with medical educators, focusing in particular on the themes that connect in important ways to the data drawn from medical students and experienced doctors.

Today, there is broad agreement that 'medical education is about more than acquiring an appropriate level of knowledge and developing relevant skills', and that, 'medicine students need to develop a professional identity', including paying attention to the ethical dimensions of medical practice (Goldie, 2012: 641). An earlier study found that, so far as integrating medical ethics within the medical school curriculum was concerned, the UK is 'ahead of the game, compared with the US and Canada ...' (Mattick and Bligh, 2006: 184). Though precisely *how* medical ethics was covered within their respective programmes differed, it was clear from the interviews that medical ethics formed an important component of the curriculum of the medical schools in which respondents worked. What comes through in the interviews is a mix of official attention to medical ethics within the curriculum alongside the workings of various more informal and at times less structured educational processes through which medical students could engage with ethical issues (a pattern that was also apparent in the interviews with medical students). One medical educator, for example, spoke of the various ways that medical students engaged with the ethical during their studies, including that:

> *We do have quite a strong ethics and humanities element to the undergraduate curriculum. It is there and we promote good role models … it's taught within every module, near enough, so when we blueprinted it we could show that within every module across the five years, there was an ethical component within every aspect.*
>
> (Medical Educator)

Another medical educator also talked about the varied engagements of students with ethics during their studies, explaining that:

> *I think in years one and two, we do the lectures and that's a bit like the rules … they like those because they're the rules and in a way, they're a good starting place … but I think really what helps them reflect and really sort of try to develop the character traits that we want is actually the work that's done in the small group sessions, because we try to put a few conflicting things together, rather than just you simply follow the rules and I think that's where the real learning happens, not really in the lectures. Okay, they need to know the rules, but I think the real learning goes on in the small group sessions.*
>
> (Medical Educator)

In these two extracts we can see the various ways that ethics were reported as being part of undergraduate medical education programmes, ways that came through in many of the interviews with medical educators. Crucially, these methods combine more formal teaching with the intentional educational processes provided by role models and through the dialogical space of small group discussion sessions. These latter methods were, however, directed in particular ways. One medical educator, for example, spoke about their aim that:

> *Students can clarify for themselves where they are and also to clarify their understandings of [professional virtues and values] and where the distance is between their understandings and what the profession itself is looking for, as articulated by the regulator. So, that's how I approach that question first and foremost, by actually suspending*

judgement and getting the students to articulate themselves. As part of their task of forming themselves, as opposed to being formed by the educational intervention, they are really forming themselves and to do that, they need to have a starting point that they're self-consciously aware of, so I approach it in those terms.

(Medical Educator)

Similarly, another respondent also took a non-directive approach, describing that in the medical school in which they worked:

There is space for some learning to take place in the nature of values, but it's not a prescriptive form of learning. It's more an exploratory form of learning, where the students get the opportunity to clarify their own values and to articulate them and to have the opportunity to discuss them and to explain them to other people, so that's why I said somewhat earlier on, because it's not a values curriculum, so to speak, it's not as organised as that, but I am nevertheless satisfied that there is some structure in the curriculum whereby that type of learning has a chance to take place.

(Medical Educator)

Still another referred to the importance of students discussing ethical matters with others, and to do so in small groups with an open and non-judgemental climate,[3] something that was not altogether easy:

Students ... come into medical school already constructed individuals, with preconceptions and it's important for them to try and render these explicit to themselves, so that they're aware of what their preconceptions are and to do so in a way that's not judgemental. Guidance can always be provided to students where guidance is needed, but they need to be able in a safe environment to articulate freely how they understand things and how they approach things and that can only be done in the small group setting, where there's a degree of trust. It's a very difficult thing to achieve, but when it can be achieved, it's very effective for learning, but it doesn't always happen.

(Medical Educator)

As stated above, across the interviews with medical educators, which we hope to have indicated to some level in these vignettes, it was clear (and albeit to different degrees and extents) that the integration of ethics in medical school programmes took a range of forms, from formal lectures, to observation of role models, to open dialogue in small groups and beyond. As stated in the original project report (Arthur et al., 2015) that this was so is a matter of importance given that integrating ethics across the curriculum and through different pedagogical methods is especially important from the perspective of virtue ethics. In general terms, virtue ethicists stress how moral character formation takes place through practice in a given context over time. In this context, the mode in which students and junior doctors learn is often tacit – what, exactly, professional practice amounts to is often not a matter that is stated in curriculum documents or course outcomes, but is unstated. Indeed, Hafferty and Franks hold that medical training seen in the round is a form of moral training, in which the formal curriculum only plays a small part (Hafferty and Franks, 1994: 861). Moreover, wider literature also points to the central role played by role-models in professional education in medicine (Cruess et al., 2008; Campbell et al., 2007).

A further area focused upon in the interviews with medical educators was the idea of change in medical students' character and ethics. In this regard, change was represented in two ways. First, some of the medical educators spoke of a 'desensitisation' in medical students as they progressed through their studies (see also, Hegazi and Wilson's (2013) work on moral segmentation). One of the medical educators, for example, stated that:

> *There is a lot of talk of erosion of ideals in the literature and it's undoubtedly the case that students later on in the course on average, across a year group, will tend to be much less sensitive to ethical matters than they might have been earlier on in the course, so there's a certain amount of desensitisation that goes on and a kind of levelling that takes place, whereby there's a sort of regression to a mean.*

Second, some medical educators reflected on changes in the qualities they had noticed in medical students entering their programme – changes influenced by wider perceptions of the medical profession:

> *I would say that actually our intake of medical students has changed and I think we're much more likely now than when I started here 12 years ago to get more empathetic individuals. For me, I don't think the qualities of a good doctor have changed, but I think the public perception and perhaps the perception of the medical profession, their expectations of what a good doctor is has changed, so I think within the profession, the idea of what a good doctor is has changed and also the public expect doctors to be kind to them and speak to them.*

Of course, and while not discounting these views in anyway, it should be noted that a number of authors acknowledge the difficulty of accurately assessing virtue or professionalism. Jha et al.'s (2007) systematic review of studies from the USA and the UK found that few studies are able to robustly illustrate a change in attitudes towards professionalism as a result of teaching interventions. This is due in no small part to the difficulty of constructing psychometrically rigorous measures of students' attitudes towards professionalism and their professional values, which makes it difficult to draw firm conclusions about efficacy or ethics or professionalism education (Eckles, 2005).

Conclusion

While any data obtained in relation to abstract, though applied, dilemmas comes with important caveats, the data analysed in this chapter provide some important insights into the thinking of medical professionals at the three career stages. Fundamentally, the data reported in this chapter indicates not only that a variety of considerations are at play when doctors engage with dilemmas, but also that virtue-based and rule-based reasoning often combine in complementary ways to guide their choices and reasons. When we consider the specific virtues that, according to the expert panel, are related to the reasons selected, the virtues that stand out mirror the virtues respondents associated with their own character as a doctor and with those of an ideal doctor. That this is so gives further credence to the view that the virtues of judgement, kindness, fairness and leadership lie at the core of virtuous medical practice.

To conclude this chapter, we note once again that though determined through the expert panel process, the dilemmas are of a particular kind – somewhat abstracted from the engaged realities of respondents' professional lives. As one Graduating Student stated in their interview, echoing the involved, engaged and dialogical pedagogies emphasised by medical educators:

> *I much prefer sort of a small group discussion, which is what we did a lot in first and second year and I think it's good because you come across methods, lots of other people's opinions and personality clashes, which is what you're going to come across on the wards.*

(Graduating Student)

Looking forward, and as we return to in the conclusion next, there is methodological work here to be done to determine ways that engaging research respondents with dilemmas can maintain the benefits identified in the introductions to this chapter and this book, while also better capturing the discursive and contextually embedded nature of real-life dilemmas faced by medical practitioners.

Notes

1 For more regarding the design of the situational judgement tests, see www.jubileecentre.ac.uk/professions.
2 Discussion of all six dilemmas can be found at www.jubileecentre.ac.uk/professions.
3 See The Point of Care Foundation (2018) for work in this area since this study was conducted.

Conclusion, recommendations and further research

Introduction

As stated from the outset, and as with the wider work of the Jubilee Centre, this book and the study contained within are premised on the idea that being a 'good' professional necessarily involves more than technical skills and subject knowledge. Not only does a good doctor appreciate and embrace the ethical dimensions of their role – they also understand the various actors, policies, practices and pressures that impact on how these ethical dimensions are shaped, negotiated and enacted. Moreover, and particularly at early stages of their careers, doctors need support to understand and discuss the full gamut of the ethical aspects of their work. One could argue that all aspects of clinical work have an ethical dimension, as they involve the interpretation and synthesis of various sources of knowledge in order to do the best (often among different visions of 'the best') for another human being. Doctors, as with other professionals, work in increasingly challenging times and there are many competing demands placed upon them; medicine is fraught with complexity and uncertainty. In such contexts, the development of professional judgement and practical wisdom alongside relational forms of care are crucial. This latter statement is not to suggest that doctors should operate as autonomous individuals, though there may be times when this may occur. Rather, doctors form part of medical communities, working with other healthcare professionals and, when appropriate, patients and their families/carers.

In the preceding two chapters, various aspects of this ethical role have been explored from the perspectives of doctors across the three career stages – first-year undergraduates, graduating students and experienced doctors. In this closing chapter we draw together the overall findings from the *Virtuous Medical Practice* project, before offering several recommendations and identifying some fertile areas in need of further research.

DOI: 10.4324/9781003137887-6

Overall findings

Here we present, adapt and extend the findings of the main project report of the virtuous medical practice study (Arthur et al., 2015a: 5):

- Doctors recognise and appreciate the ethical nature of their work. Respondents across the three career stages were in substantial agreement on the virtues that doctors should possess:
  - Fairness
  - Honesty
  - Judgement
  - Kindness
  - Leadership
  - Teamwork
- Doctors in the study spoke of the positives of their working environment, being largely positive about their emotional involvement with their work and the autonomy they were afforded. Crucially, a significant aspect that sustains the ethical work of doctors is the support they gain from colleagues and, also, their families.
- In the interviews, doctors spoke of the influence of positive role models in their initial education and subsequent practice. In speaking about the importance of this learning, the doctors in the study painted a picture of the role of the culture of workplace environments, emphasising the importance of the informal curriculum and informal learning, including through observing and learning from role-models. These were seen to be significant in shaping a doctor's early professional identity.
- Doctors and medical educators reported a variety of formal ways that medical ethics is attended to within the curricular of medical schools alongside the workings of more informal and at times less structured educational processes. In addition, differences were noted in the way in which medical educators approached medical ethics, with some, for example, emphasising a non-directive approach through which medical students clarify their own values and emerging professional identity.

Overall recommendations

With these overall findings in mind, we draw on and extend on the recommendations contained within the original project report (Arthur, 2015a) to propose the following overall recommendations:

- Literacy in the language of character and virtue needs to be included in the formal curriculum of initial medical education and training, including paying intentional attention for how character and virtue are experienced and learned through informal interactions with experienced doctors. Embracing a variety of ethical theories – including how these cohere (or otherwise) in practice, will help medical students to make sense of, understand and reflect upon the ethical dimensions of medical practice. This would include insight into how the rules-based ethical frameworks that dominate healthcare and medical education play a part within a virtue ethics approach.

- In order to make sense, understand and reflect upon the ethical dimensions of medical practice, doctors at various stages of their career need the time, space and opportunity to come together (in small groups, for example) to discuss real-life ethical quandaries and the potential responses. Such time, space and opportunities are particularly crucial for medical students and doctors at an early stage of their careers. It remains important to determine the enablers and barriers to this work.

- It is clear that role-modelling and the culture within the environments in which doctors work influence the learning and professional development of doctors at an early stage of their career. Given this, more attention needs to be paid to informal education in moral character, and those responsible for medical education should create more opportunities for early career doctors to engage with experienced others to reflect on ethics in the workplace. Medical educators need to realise how powerful role models, informal learning and the hidden curriculum are when it comes to nurturing virtues and values. Educators need also to appreciate their role in influencing learners in the development of virtue.

Future research

The analysis of data presented in this book raises a myriad of possible trajectories and emphases for future research. To extend current understandings of what constitutes 'the good doctor' the following are particularly relevant:

- Noting the presence of studies published since the *Virtuous Medical Practice* study concluded (for example, Conroy et al., 2021 and Jameel, 2021) further research is needed that examines the professional wisdom of doctors, including how this wisdom is mediated, negotiated and enacted in practice.

- While the data analysed in the project and reported in this book focused on doctors at particular stages of their professional career, further longitudinal research tracking the same doctor(s) over a sustained period of time are likely to obtain a deeper sense of the trajectories and nuances of being a 'good' doctor, including the ethical dimensions of the profession. This would help determine if the virtues are stable traits or not. Looking more specifically at *phronesis*, longitudinal studies would enable insight into how this meta-virtue is developed throughout a doctor's career.
- While the study reported here drew on responses to moral dilemmas as a research instrument, as we have noted these are not without their limitations. Further work on different ways of understanding and measuring doctors' handling of complex moral quandaries are needed.
- Similar to other studies, the medical educators involved in the *Virtuous Medical Practice* project presented a mixed and diverse picture of how medical ethics featured within their curricular. While medical ethics should not be reduced to a singular, universal approach there remains a need for further research that sheds light on excellence in this area, and which enables the work of leading medical educators in this area to be shared more widely. It is also worth considering if education on professional virtues sits better across professional education rather than in discrete ethics modules.
- The interplay between developing the virtues and the role/impact of organisational culture needs further exploration. It is clear from this research that work environments and educational institutions have a large part to play nurturing virtues in context. Organisations and institutions need to realise the importance of orchestrating the climate that enables clinicians to flourish, and we need to know more about how this can and does occur.

References

Adams, P. (2009) 'Ethics with character: Virtues and the ethical social worker', *The Journal of Sociology & Social Welfare*, 36(3), pp. 83–105.

Andah, E., Essang, B., Friend, C., Greenley, S., Harvey, K., Spears, M., and Reeve, J. (2021) 'Understanding the impact of professional motivation on the workforce crisis in medicine: a rapid review', *BJGP Open*, DOI:10.3399/BJGPO.2021.0005.

Arthur, J., Kristjánsson, K., Thomas, H., Holdsworth, M., Badini Confolonieri, L., and Qiu, T. (2014) *Virtuous Character for the Practice of Law: Research Report*. Birmingham: Jubilee Centre for Character and Virtues, University of Birmingham.

Arthur, J., Kristjánsson, K., Thomas, H., Kotzee, B., Ignatowicz, A., and Qiu, T. (2015a) *Virtuous Medical Practice*. Jubilee Centre for Character and Virtues.

Arthur, J., Kristjánsson, K., Cooke, S., Brown, E., and Carr, D. (2015b) *The Good Teacher: Understanding Virtues in Practice*. Jubilee Centre for Character and Virtues.

Arthur, J., Earl, S., Thompson, A., and Ward, J. (2019a) *Repurposing the Professions: The Role of Professional Character – Initial Insights*. Jubilee Centre for Character and Virtues.

Arthur, J., Earl, S. R., Thompson, A. P., and Ward, J. W. (2019b) 'The value of character-based judgement in the professional domain', *Journal of Business Ethics*, DOI: 10.1007/s10551-019-04269-7.

Arthur, J., Walker, D. I., and Thoma, S. J. (2018) *Soldiers of Character: Research Report*. Birmingham: Jubilee Centre for Character and Virtues, University of Birmingham.

Ashcroft, R., Baron, D., and Benatar, S. (1998) 'Teaching Medical Ethics and Law Within Medical Education: A Model for the UK Core Curriculum', *Journal of Medical Ethics*, 24(3), pp. 188–192.

Barilan, Y. M. and Brusa, M. (2012) 'Deliberation at the hub of medical education: beyond virtue ethics and codes of practice', *Medicine, Health Care and Philosophy*, 16(1), pp. 1–10.

Beauchamp, T. and Childress, J. (1979) *Principles of Biomedical Ethics*. Oxford: Oxford University Press.

Berwick, D. M. (2016) 'Era 3 for medicine and health care', *JAMA*, 315(13), pp. 1329–1330.

Bessant, J. (2009) 'Aristotle meets youth work: A case for virtue ethics', *Journal of Youth Studies*, 12(4), pp. 423–438.

Blendon, R. J., Benson, J. M., and Hero, J. M. (2014) 'Public trust in physicians – U.S. medicine in international perspective', *The New England Journal of Medicine*, 371(17), pp. 1570–1572.

Blond, P., Antonacopoulou, E., and Pabst, A. (2015) *In Professions We Trust: Fostering Virtuous Practitioners in Teaching, Law and Medicine.* London: Respublica.

Bohlin, K. (2005) *Teaching Character Education Through Literature: Awakening the Moral Imagination in Secondary Classrooms.* London: Routledge.

Bontemps-Hommen, C. M. M. L., Baart, A., and Vosman, F. T. H. (2019) 'Practical wisdom in complex medical practices: A critical proposal', *Medicine, Health-Care and Philosophy*, 22, 95–105.

Borgstrom, E., Cohn, S., and Barclay, S. (2010) 'Medical professionalism: conflicting values for tomorrow's doctors', *Journal of General Internal Medicine*, 25(12), pp. 1330–1336.

British Broadcasting Corporation (2017) Online GP consultation of 'limited use', study finds, www.bbc.co.uk/news/uk-england-42084224 [accessed 21 May 2021].

Brody, H. and Doukas, D. (2014) 'Professionalism: A framework to guide medical education', *Medical Education*, 48(10), pp. 980–987.

Bruce, D. A. (2007) 'Regulation of doctors', *British Medical Journal*, 334(37), pp. 433–434.

Bryan, C. and Babelay, A. (2009) 'Building character: A model for reflective practice', *Academic Medicine*, 84(9), pp. 1283–1288.

Campbell, D. (2021) 'GPs prefer to see patients face to face, says UK family doctors' leader', 28 March, *The Guardian*, www.theguardian.com/society/2021/mar/28/gps-prefer-to-see-patients-face-to-face-says-uk-family-doctors-leader

Campbell, A., Chin, J., and Voo, T-C. (2007) 'How can we know that ethics education produces ethical doctors?', *Medical Teacher*, 29(5), pp. 431–436.

Campbell, A. V. and Chin, J. J. (2011) 'Preserving medical ethics and professionalism: Meeting the challenges of modern practice', *Annals of the Academy of Medicine, Singapore*, Jan, 40(1), pp. 1–3. PMID: 21369626.

Cardenas, D. (2020) 'Surgical ethics: a framework for surgeons, patients, and society', *Bioethics in Surgery*, 47, pp. 1–10.

Carr, D. (1999) 'Professional education and professional ethics', *Journal of Applied Philosophy*, 16(1), pp. 33–46.

Carr, D. (2011) 'Virtue, character and emotion in people professions: Towards a virtue ethics of interpersonal professional conduct', in Bondi, L., Carr, D., Clark, C., and Clegg, C. (eds.) *Towards Professional Wisdom: Practical Deliberation in the People Professions.* Farnham: Ashgate.

Carr, D. (2018) 'Introduction', in Carr, D. (ed.) *Cultivating Moral Character and Virtue in Professional Practice.* Abingdon: Routledge, pp. 1–12.

Charles, A. (2015) 'Do the public still trust doctors and nurses?', www.kingsfund.org.uk/blog/2015/12/public-trust-doctors-nurses; accessed 4 April 2021.

Christmas, S. and Millward, L. (2011) *New Medical Professionalism: A Scoping Report for the Health Foundation.* London: The Health Foundation.

Conroy, M., Malik, A. Y., Hale, C., Weir, C., Brockie, A., and Turner, C. (2021) 'Using practical wisdom to facilitate ethical decision-making: a major empirical study of *phronesis* in the decision narratives of doctors', *BMC Medical Ethics*, 22, 16. https://doi.org/10.1186/s12910-021-00581-y.

Cooke, S. and Carr, D. (2014) 'Virtue, practical wisdom and character in teaching', *British Journal of Educational Studies*, 62(2), 91–110.

Coulehan, J. (2005) 'Today's professionalism: Engaging the mind but not the heart', *Academic Medicine*, 80(10), pp. 892–898.

Cruess, S., Cruess, R., and Steinert, Y. (2008) 'Role modelling – making the most of a powerful teaching strategy', *British Medical Journal*, 336, pp. 718–721.

Cruess, S. R., Johnston, S., and Cruess, R. L. (2004) '"Profession": A working definition for medical educators', *Teaching and Learning in Medicine*, 16(1), 74–76.

Department of Health (2001) Learning from Bristol: The Report of the Public Inquiry Into Children's Heart Surgery at the Bristol Royal Infirmary 1984–1995 (Cm 5363). London: The Stationary Office.

Dixon-Woods, M., Yeung, K., and Bosk, C. L. (2011) 'Why is UK medicine no longer a self-regulating profession? The role of scandals involving "bad apple" doctors', *Social Science & Medicine*, 73(10), pp. 1452–1459.

Dowie, A. (2000) 'Phronesis or "practical wisdom" in medical education', *Medical Teacher*, 22(3), 240–241.

Eckles, R., Meslin, E., Gaffney, M., and Helft, P. (2005) 'Medical ethics education: Where are we? Where should we be going? A review', *Academic Medicine*, 80(12), pp. 1143–1152.

Editorial (2020) *British Journal of Oral and Maxillofacial Surgery*, 58, pp. 125–128.

Elledge, R. and Jones, J. (2020) 'Character failings in the surgeon fallen from grace: a thematic analysis of disciplinary hearings against surgeons 2016–2020', *Journal of Medical Ethics*. DOI: 10.1136/medethics-2020-106809.

Ericsson, K. A., Charness, N., Feltovich, P. J., and Hoffman, R. R. (eds.). (2006) *The Cambridge Handbook of Expertise and Expert Performance.* Cambridge University Press.

Eurofund (2012) *5th Eurofund Working Conditions Survey.* Luxembourg: Publications Office of the European Union.

Field, R. (2008) 'Why is health care regulation so complex?', *Pharmacy and Therapeutics*, 33(10), pp. 607–608.

Fish, D. and de Cossart, L. (2013) *Reflection for Medical Appraisal: Exploring and Developing Your Clinical Expertise and Professional Identity.* Gloucester: Aneumi Publications.

Furlong, W., Crossan, M., Gandz, J., and Crossan, I. (2017) 'Character's essential role in addressing misconduct in financial institutions', *Business Law International*, 18, p. 199.

Gardiner, P. (2003) 'A virtue ethics approach to moral dilemmas in medicine', *Journal of Medical Ethics*, 29(5), 297–302.

Gawande, A. (2011) *The Checklist Manifesto: How to Get Things Right*. London: Profile Books.

General Medical Council (1993) *Tomorrow's Doctors: Recommendations on Undergraduate Medical Education*. London: General Medical Council.

General Medical Council (2017) *Generic Professional Capabilities Framework*. Manchester: General Medical Council.

General Medical Council (2018) *Outcomes for Graduates*. Manchester: General Medical Council.

General Medical Council (2019) *Good Medical Practice*, www.gmc-uk.org/ethical-guidance/ethical-guidance-for-doctors/good-medical-practice [accessed 23 May 2021].

Gillies, J. (2005) 'Getting it right in the consultation: Hippocrates's problems, Aristotle's solution'. Occasional Paper 86. RGCP.

Glaser, B. G. and Strauss, A. L. (1967) *The Discovery of Grounded Theory: Strategies for Qualitative Research*. Chicago: Aldine.

Goldie, J. (2012) 'The formation of professional identity in medical students: Considerations for educators', *Medical Teacher*, 34(9), pp. 641–648.

Great Britain. Parliament. House of Commons (2013) Report of the Mid Staffordshire NHS Foundation Trust Public Inquiry by Francis, R., London: The Stationery Office (HC 2012–2013 898–1).

Hafferty, F. and Franks, R. (1994) 'The hidden curriculum: Ethics teaching, and the structure of medical education', *Academic Medicine*, 69(11), pp. 861–871.

Hall, D. (2001) 'Reflecting on Redfern: What can we learn from the Alder Hey story?', *Archives of Disease in Childhood*, 84(6), pp. 455–456.

Hannah, M. (2014) *Humanising Healthcare: Patterns of Hope for a System Under Strain*. Devon: Triarchy Press.

Harrison, T. and Khatoon, B. (2017) *Virtue, Practical Wisdom and Professional Education: A Pilot Intervention Designed to Enhance Virtue Knowledge, Understanding and Reasoning in Student Lawyers, Doctors and Teachers*. Jubilee Centre for Character and Virtues.

Heath, I. (2015) 'Arm in arm with righteousness', *Philosophy, Ethics, and Humanities in Medicine*, 10(1), p. 7.

Hegazi, I. and Wilson, I. (2013) 'Medical education and moral segmentation in medical students', *Medical Education*, 47(10), pp. 1022–1028.

Hilton, S. and Slotnick, H. (2005) 'Proto-professionalism: How professionalisation occurs across the continuum of medical education', *Medical Education*, 39(1), pp. 58–65.

Hilton, S. and Southgate, L. (2007) 'Professionalism in medical education', *Teaching and Teacher Education*, 23, pp. 265–279.

Holbeche, L. and Springett, N. (2004) *'In Search of Meaning at Work'*, Roffey Park Institute, Horsham, http://citeseerx.ist.psu.edu/viewdoc/download?doi=10.1.1.458.1538&rep=rep1&type=pdf [accessed 18 May 2018].

Huang, E., C-H., Pu, C. P., Chou, Y-J., and Huang, N. (2018) 'Public trust in physicians – health care commodification as a possible deteriorating factor: cross-sectional analysis of 23 countries', *INQUIRY: The Journal of Health Care Organization, Provision, and Financing*, 55, 1–11.

Iles, V., Sweeney. K., and Vaughan Smith, J. (2009) 'What makes good doctors practise bad medicine?', www.reallylearning.com/Current_Projects/Learning_Sets/What_makes_good_Doctors_practise_bad_medicine2_3_09.pdf [accessed 9 April 2021].

Institute of Medical Ethics (1987) *The Pond Report: Report of a Working Party on the Teaching of Medical Ethics*, London: IME Publications.

Institute of Medical Ethics (2019) *Core Curriculum for Undergraduate Medical Ethics and Law*. London: Institute of Medical Ethics.

Ipsos MORI (2011) Trust in Professions 2011, [Online], Available: www.ipsos-mori.com/researchpublications/researcharchive/2818/Doctors-are-most-trusted-profession-politiciansleast-trusted.aspx [accessed 17 October 2014].

Ipsis Mori (2017) 'Politicians remain the least trusted profession in Britain', www.ipsos.com/ipsos-mori/en-uk/politicians-remain-least-trusted-profession-britain#:~:text=The%20Ipsos%20MORI%20Veracity%20Index,weather%20forecasters%20and%20professional%20footballers [accessed 6 April 2021].

Jameel, S. (2021) 'Wise Doctors: What can they teach us about flourishing?', *The Journal of Holistic Healthcare*, 18(1), pp. 49–52.

Jha, V., Bekker, H. L., Duffy, S. R. G., and Roberts, T. E. (2006) 'Perceptions of professionalism in medicine: a qualitative study', *Medical Education*, 40(10), pp. 1027–1036.

Jha, V., Bekker, H. L., Duffy, S. R. G., and Roberts, T. E. (2007) 'A systematic review of studies assessing and facilitating attitudes towards professionalism in medicine' [Review], *Medical Education*, 41(8), 822–829.

Jubilee Centre for Character and Virtues (2017) *A Framework for Character Education in Schools*. University of Birmingham, Jubilee Centre for Character and Virtues, www.jubileecentre.ac.uk/userfiles/jubileecentre/pdf/character-education/Framework%20for%20Character%20Education.pdf [accessed 14 August 2019].

Kassam, K. A. (2010) 'Practical wisdom and ethical awareness through student experiences of development', *Development in Practice*, 20(2), pp. 205–218.

Kinghorn, W. A. (2010) 'Medical Education as Moral Formation. An Aristotelian account of medical professionalism', *Perspectives in Biology and Medicine*, 53(1), pp. 87–105.

Kinsella, E. A. and Pitman, A. (2012) 'Engaging phronesis in professional practice and education', in E. A. Kinsella and A. Pitman (eds.) *Phronesis as Professional Knowledge: Practical Wisdom in the Professions*. Rotterdam: Sense, pp. 1–13.

Kladjian, L. C. (2010) 'Teaching practical wisdom in medicine through clinical judgement, goals of care and ethical reasoning', *Journal of Medical Ethics*, 36(9), pp. 558–562.

Kotzee, B., Paton, A., and Conroy, M. (2016) 'Towards an empirically informed account of *phronesis* in medicine', *Perspectives in Biology and Medicine*, 59(3), pp. 337–350.

Kristjánsson, K. (2015a) 'Phronesis as an ideal in professional medical ethics: Some preliminary positionings and problematics', *Theoretical Medicine and Bioethics*, 36(5), 299–320.

Kristjánsson, K. (2015b) *Aristotelian Character Education*. Abingdon: Routledge.

Kristjánsson, K., Arthur, J., Moller, F., and Huo, Y. (2017a) *Character and Virtues In Business and Finance*. Jubilee Centre for Character and Virtues.

Kristjánsson, K., Varghese, J., Arthur, J., and Moller, F. with Ferkany, M. (2017b) *Virtuous Practice in Nursing*. Jubilee Centre for Character and Virtues.

Kristjánsson, K., Thomas, H., Kotzee, B., Ignatowicz, A., and Qiu, T. (2015) *Virtuous Medical Practice*. Jubilee Centre for Character and Virtues.

Larkin, G. L., Iserson, K., Kassutto, Z., Freas, G., Delaney, K., Krimm, J., … Adams, J. (2009) "Virtue in emergency medicine", *Academic Emergency Medicine*, 16(1), pp. 51–55.

Lehman, R. (2017) 'Sharing as the Future of Medicine', *JAMA Internal Medicine*, 177(9), pp. 1237–1238.

Lewis, C. S. (1985) *Letters to Children*, New York: MacMillan.

Lievens, F. and Patterson, F. (2011) 'The validity and incremental validity of knowledge tests, low-fidelity simulations and high-fidelity simulations for predicting job performance in advanced-level high-stakes selection', *Journal of Applied Psychology*, 96(5), pp. 927–940.

Mattick, K. and Bligh, J. (2006) 'Teaching and assessing medical ethics: Where are we now?', *Journal of Medical Ethics*, 32(3), pp. 181–185.

McDougall, R. (2013) 'Understanding doctors' ethical challenges as role virtue conflicts', *Bioethics*, 27(1), 20–27.

McKie, A., Baguley, F., Guthrie, C., Jackson, C., Kirkpatrick, P., Laing, A., O'Brien, S., Taylor, R., and Wimpenny, P. (2012) 'Exploring clinical wisdom in nursing education', *Nursing Ethics*, 19(2), pp. 252–267.

McKinley, N., McCain, R., Convie, L., Clarke, M., Dempster, M., Campbell, W., and Kirk, S. (2020) 'Resilience, burnout and coping mechanisms in UK doctors: A cross-sectional study', *BMJ Open*, 10(1), pp. e031765.

Montori, V. (2017) *Why We Revolt: A Patient Revolution for Careful and Kind Care*. Missouri: The Patient Revolution.

Moore, G. (2015) 'Corporate character, corporate virtues', *Business Ethics: A European Review*, 24(2), pp. 99–114.

Oakley, J. and Cocking, D. (2001) *Virtue Ethics and Professional Roles*. Cambridge: Cambridge University Press.

Office for Standards in Education (2019) *Teacher Well-being at Work in Schools and Further Education Providers*, https://assets.publishing.service.gov.uk/government/uploads/system/uploads/attachment_data/file/819314/Teacher_well-being_report_110719F.pdf [accessed 9 September 2019].

Ong, Y. T., Kow, C. S., Teo, Y. H., Tan, L. H. E., Abdurrahman, A. B. H. M, Quek, N. W. S., Prakash, K., Cheong, C. W. S., Tan, X. H., Lim, W. Q., Wu,

J., Tan, L. H. S., Tay, K. T., Chin, A., Toh, Y. P., Mason, S., and Krishna, L. K. R. (2020) 'Nurturing professionalism in medical schools. A systematic scoping review of training curricula between 1990–2019', *Medical Teacher*, 42(6), 636–649.

Paes, P., Leat, D., and Stewart, J. (2018) 'Complex decision making in medical training: key internal and external influences in developing pratical wisdom', *Clinical Reasoning*, 53, pp. 165–174.

Paterson, R. (2013) *The Good Doctor: What Patients Want*. Auckland: Auckland University Press.

Paton, A. and Kotzee, B. (2019) 'The fundamental role of storytelling and practical wisdom in facilitating the ethics education of junior doctors', *Health*, pp. 1–17.

Patterson, F. and Ashworth, V. (2011) *Situational Judgement Tests: The Future of Medical selection?*, [Online], Available at: http://careers.bmj.com/careers/advice/view-article.html?id=20005183 [accessed 2 April 2021].

Pellegrino, E. D. (1995) 'Toward a vitue-based normative ethics for the health-professions', *Kennedy Institute of Ethics Journal*, 5(3), 253–277.

Pellegrino, E. and Thomasma, D. (1993) *The Virtues in Medical Practice*. Oxford: Oxford University Press.

Peterson, C. and Seligman, M. (2004) *Character Strengths and Virtues: A Handbook and Classification*. Oxford: Oxford University Press.

Pitman, A. (2012) 'Professionalism and professionalization: Hostile ground for growing phronesis', in E. A. Kinsella and A. Pitman (eds.) *Phronesis as Professional Knowledge: Practical Wisdom in the Professions*. Rotterdam: Sense, pp. 131–146.

Point of Care Foundation (2018) *Audit of the Teaching of Professionalism in Undergraduate Medical Education*, www.pointofcarefoundation.org.uk/resource/audit-of-the-teaching-of-professionalism-in-undergraduate-medical-education/ [accessed 1 April 2021].

Rhodes, R. (2020) *The Trusted Doctor: Medical Ethics and Professionalism*. Oxford: Oxford University Press.

Richie, J. and Spencer, L. (1994) 'Qualitative data analysis for applied policy research', in Bryman, A. and Burgess, B. (eds.) *Analysing Qualitative Data*. London: Routledge.

Rodriguez-Jareño, M. C., Demou, E., Vargas-Prada, S., Sanati, K. A., Škerjanc, A., Reis, P. G., Helimäki-Aro, R., Macdonald, E. B., and Serra, C. (2014) European Working Time Directive and doctors' health: A systematic review of the available epidemiological evidence. *BMJ Open*, 4: e004916. doi:10.1136/ bmjopen-2014-004916

Royal Pharmaceutical Society (2011) *Reducing Workplace Pressure Through Professional Empowerment*. www.rpharms.com/Portals/0/RPS%20document%20library/Open%20access/Support/64585_Reducing%20Workplace%20Pressure%20through%20professional%20empowerment%20-%20FINAL. PDF?ver=2017-05-16-133220-000, accessed 20 November 2019.

Russell, D. (2009) *Practical Intelligence and the Virtues*. Oxford: Oxford University Press.

Ruzycki, S. M., Traboulsi, D., and Stanley-Bhanji, S. (2018) 'Empathy and transactional medicine: Improving patient and physician outcomes', in *Practical Dermatology*. November. 74–77.

Salisbury, H. (2020) 'Is transactional care enough?', *BMJ*, https://doi.org/10.1136/bmj.m226.

Schultz, D. S. and Carnevale, F. A. (1996) 'Engagement and suffering in responsible caregiving: On overcoming maleficence in health care', *Theoretical Medicine*, 17(3), pp. 189–207.

Schwartz, B. (2009) 'Our loss of wisdom', *TED2009*. www.ted.com/talks/barry_schwartz_our_loss_of_wisdom?; accessed 24 November 2019.

Schwartz, B. (2011) 'Using our practical wisdom', *TEDSalon New York*. www.ted.com/talks/barry_schwartz_using_our_practical_wisdom?language=en, accessed 24 November 2019.

Schwartz, B. and Sharpe, K. (2010) *Practical Wisdom: The Right Way to Do the Right Thing*. New York: Riverhead Books.

Seijts, G., Crossan, M., and Carleton, E. (2017) 'Embedding leader character into HR practices and to achieve sustained excellence', *Organizational Dynamics*, 44(1), 65–74.

Sellman, D. (2009) 'Practical wisdom in health and social care: Teaching for professional phronesis', *Learning in Health and Social Care*, 8(2), pp. 84–91.

Sellman, D. (2012) 'Reclaiming competence for professional phronesis', in E. A. Kinsella and A. Pitman (eds.) *Phronesis as Professional Knowledge: Practical Wisdom in the Professions*. Rotterdam: Sense, pp. 115–130.

Serodio, A., Kopelman, B., and Bataglia, P. (2016) 'The promotion of medical students' moral development: A comparison between a traditional course on bioethics and a course complemented with the Konstanz method of dilemma discussion', *International Journal of Ethics Education*, 1(1), pp. 81–89.

Stenersen Hovdenak, S. and Wiese, E. F. (2018) 'Promoting professional development in medical education: Persepectives from the Norwegian medical school in Tromsoe', *Society, Health & Vulnerability*, 9(1), pp. 1–10.

Tallis, R. (2006) 'Doctors in society: Medical professionalism in a changing world', *Clinical Medicine*, 6(1), pp. 7–12.

The Independent (2013) 'The Francis Report: The Key Findings', www.independent.co.uk/life-style/health-and-families/health-news/francis-report-key-findings-8484071.html [accessed 2 April 2021].

Toon, P. D. (2014) *A Flourishing Practice?* London: RGCP.

Veatch, R. M. (2006) 'Character formation in professional education: A word of caution', in Kenny, N., and Shelton, W. (eds.) *Lost Virtue: Professional Character Development in Medical Ethics*. Amsterdam: Elsevier.

Walker, F. O. (2005) 'Essay – Cultivating simple virtues in medicine', *Neurology*, 65(10), pp. 1678–1680.

West, A. (2017) 'The ethics of professional accountants: An Aristotelian perspective', *Accounting, Auditing & Accountability Journal*, 30(2), 328–351.

West, M. and Coia, D. (2019) *Caring for Doctors, Caring for Patients.* www.gmc-uk.org/-/media/documents/caring-for-doctors-caring-for-patients_pdf-80706341.pdf.

Worth, J. and Van Den Brande, J. (2019) *Teacher Labour Market in England: Annual Report 2019*, www.nfer.ac.uk/media/3344/teacher_labour_market_in_england_2019.pdf [accessed 20 November 2019].

Index